Dr. Del's 10 Minute™ Meals

Quick & Easy Recipes for Building a Lean and Healthy Body

A simple way to develop your own personalized meal plan to build a fit, lean and sexy body.

How to make healthy delicious meals that taste great in less than ten minutes!

How to make healthy meals that you will enjoy eating regularly without sacrificing taste and flavor!

Over 130 quick and easy 10-minute recipes that will help you to build muscle and lose fat (vegetarian recipes included)!

Del Millers, PhD

Dr. Del's 10 Minute Meals
Quick and Easy Recipes for Building a Lean and Healthy Body

Del Millers, Ph.D.

Published by

Spiritwind Publications
10736 Jefferson Blvd., # 693
Culver City, CA 90230 U.S.A.
888-800-9463

Publisher's Cataloging-in-Publication Data
Millers, Del.
Dr. Del's 10 Minute Meals: Quick & Easy Recipes for
Building a lean and Healthy Body / Del Millers. -- 1st ed.
p. cm.

ISBN 978-0-9856443-7-6
1. Nutrition 2. Quick and easy cookery.
I. Title.
RA784.M55 2003 613.2
QB102-200700

Design by Linda B & Dotti Albertine
Photographs Michael Burr Photography

Printed in the United States of America

"If you eat crap, you will look and feel like crap!"
~ Del Millers

When I despair,
I remember that all through history
the way of truth and love has always won.
There have been tyrants and murderers
and for a time they seem invincible,
but in the end, they always fall—think of it ALWAYS.

MAHATMA GANDHI

WHAT OTHERS ARE SAYING

"This isn't just another recipe book; this is a complete nutrition guide. You'll learn what to eat, when to eat, how much to eat and get all your fitness and nutrition questions answered as well. This book is an invaluable resource."

— **Marilyn Joyce, MA, RD, Ph.D. (c)**
Author, *5 Minutes to Health*
Author, *I Can't Believe It's Tofu*

"I love Del's recipes. They're simple, healthy and delicious."

— **Lauren Dillard, MD**
San Diego, CA

"This is a great nutrition guide. I'm going to recommend it to all my clients."

— **Mike Kaplan**
Personal Trainer

"In one simple book, I've learned how to shop, what to cook, and what supplements to take. Thank you! Thank you!"

— **Dotti Albertine**
Albertine Graphic Design

"Del has been my personal chef for many years. He's a master at making healthy food that tastes great!"

— **Andrew Hawley**
Los Angeles, CA

"This is a great book because it helps me to understand what I should eat before, during and after my workouts. I also like how easy Del made it for me to calculate how many calories I should be eating daily and what foods I should eat."

— **Jenny Leone, Model**

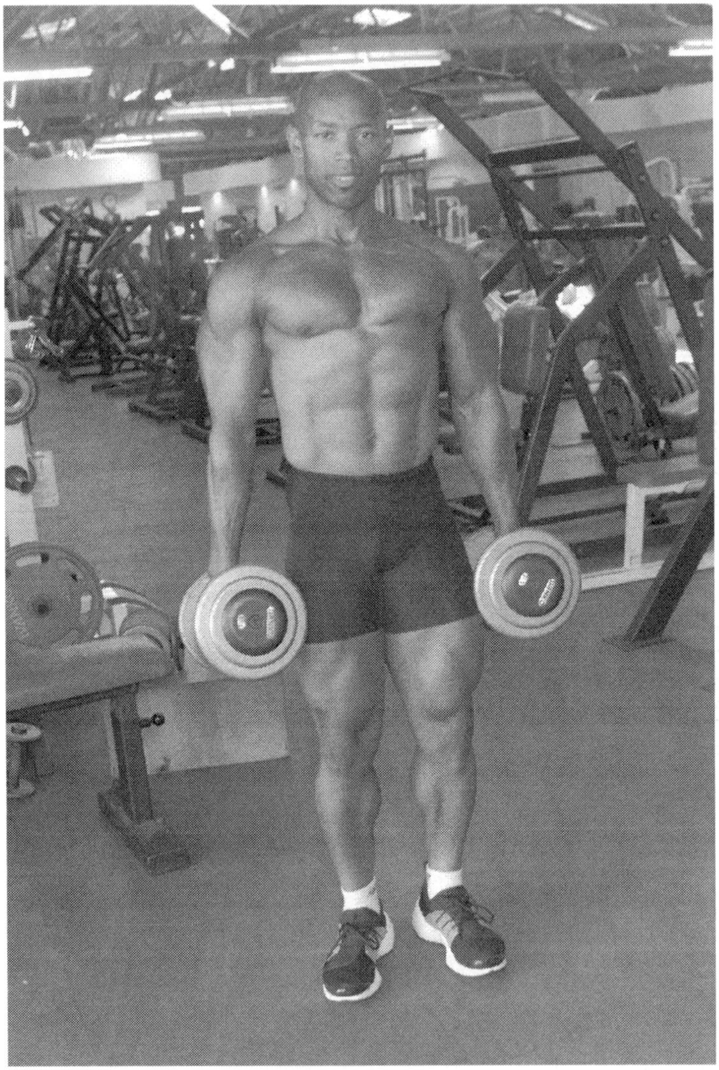

It isn't enough to be inspired.

You've got to take action.

— Del Millers

C O N T E N T S

TO THE READER

HERE IS THE MOST IMPORTANT MESSAGE TO GET FROM THIS BOOK:

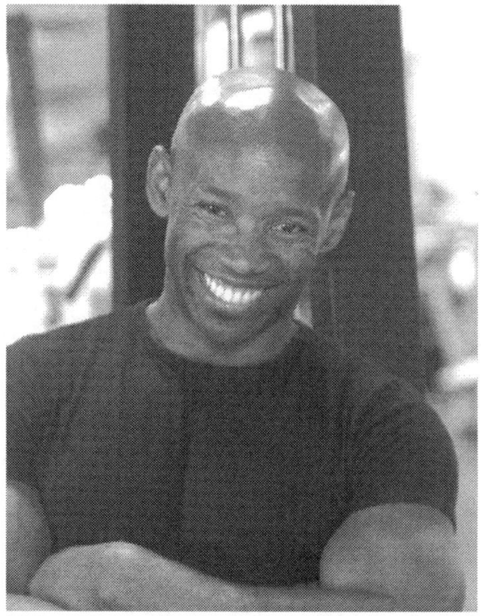

You will never change your body without practicing good nutritional habits consistently…No matter how hard or how often you exercise!

- Food is the key to radiant health and a great-looking body.
- Food is the biggest difference between those who look great and those who don't!
- With good nutrition, you will feel vibrant, energetic and alive.

With good nutrition, you will recover faster from illness or injury. Without good nutrition, you will feel lethargic, depressed, unmotivated, tired and sickly!

PERIOD!

GOOD NUTRITION IS THE KEY!

You are what you eat, that's easy to say
But if you want a healthy body, there's no other way
Eat right, clear your mind, get an exercise plan
Been this way since time began
It's the same for every woman and man

Yeah you are what you eat, that's easy to say
So when you gonna start; how 'bout today?

You've heard the phrase, "you are what you eat." How many of us realize the literal meaning of those words?

Think with me for a second. Every organ and tissue in your body (heart, liver, kidney, brain, muscle, skin, etc.) is made of microscopic cells. And where does your body get the raw material to build those cells?

If your answer is FOOD, you've hit the lettuce right on the head. Make no mistake about it, ***the foods we eat today we wear tomorrow***. This can either be in the form of beautiful rippling muscles, soft radiant skin and healthy functioning organs, or it can look like obesity, acne, heart disease, cancer, hypertension, arthritis, and a host of other diseases — all of which can be prevented with good nutrition!

The choice is yours, so choose wisely!

You've already started to make good choices. You've chosen this book. Congratulations, this means that you're interested in good nutrition. (Unless you got this book from your mate or your mother, in which case *they* would like for you to learn nutrition. I bet you know why!) With this in mind, I have carefully created or selected each recipe that I think is not only *simple* and *delicious,* but also very *healthy* and *nutritious.*

ENJOY!
Del Millers

WHY ARE WE STILL FAT?

I should look super
I work out like a trooper
And I burn burn burn
None of my hard work shows
So I still yearn yearn yearn
To get into my favorite clothes
When will I learn learn learn
It's not just pounding up the street
Or aerobicizing to a jungle beat
It's also what you eat
Gotta watch what you eat

I see you at the gym, I see you walking almost every day, I see you on the treadmill for — what looks to be — hours at a time. Here's a question for you. How is it that you seem to spend all your free time either sweating in the gym, plodding on the running trail, or working out at home, and you still don't look the way you want?

For all your effort, you should be a fitness magazine model. Instead, you're still struggling to fit into your favorite outfit.

Here's the bitter truth: your problem isn't the exercise. The problem is with your nutrition program.

80% of changing your body is nutrition related.

The Body Transformation Program and recipes in this book have already helped hundreds of my personal clients and seminar participants get the results they're looking for. You're no exception. But first, you must follow a nutrition plan. I have outlined one for you in this book. All you have to do is follow it.

Let me repeat that. To get the results you want, *you have* to *follow the plan* in this book, not just read about it!

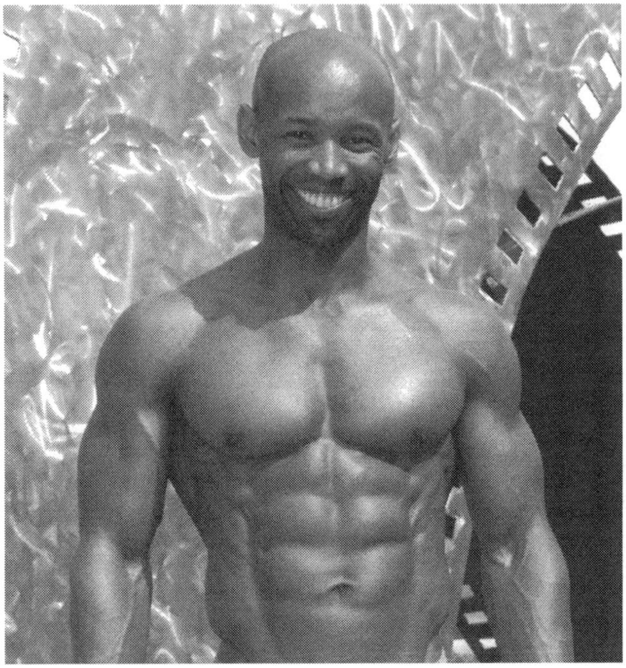

"If you don't eat the right foods,
you will end up wearing the wrong ones!"
— Del Millers

NUTRITION, DISEASE AND PREVENTION

▼ HERE'S SOMETHING FOR YOU TO THINK ABOUT:

Each minute, 300 million of your body cells die! And others are created to take their place. Of course, some cells last for years and others divide every day through a process called Mitosis. Normally, genes are duplicated within the original cell before that cell divides. Sometimes, however, they are not duplicated exactly. These inexact copies are called ***genetic mutations*** *and become part of the genetic code of subsequent cells.*

What contributes to genetic mutation? Environmental carcinogens (smoking, toxic air, etc.), heredity, lack of necessary building materials (poor nutritional habits), free radical damage, mutations in the "P53" Protein. (Called the "Guardian of the Genome," P53 prevents cells from going through mitosis with damaged DNA.)

In a nutshell, poor nutrition and a shaky lifestyle causes our cells to mutate with inaccurate genetic information. Ultimately, these cells become cancerous or lead to other diseases such as heart disease, diabetes, arthritis, and other immune deficiency conditions — you get the picture.

How do we prevent this from happening? Here's the simple part! Just give the body what it needs and it will take care of the rest. You must eat a variety of fruits and vegetables of all different colors, as well as grains, legumes (beans and peas) and lean protein. We don't yet have a cure for cancer, heart disease, diabetes and other chronic diseases, but we do know for a fact that the right balance of good nutrition can dramatically reduce your chances of getting them by over 50%!

▼ BASIC CONCEPTS OF ENERGY (FOOD) METABOLISM

One of the reasons that many people abuse their bodies with food and improper exercise is because they just don't understand how the body works. For instance, how does your body convert the foods you eat into usable energy for your working muscles? If you don't really know the answer, don't feel bad, this area of energy metabolism and exercise physiology is very complicated. However, I think it is important to understand, especially if you are an athlete or avid exerciser. So I will simplify it for you.

▼ THE THREE ENERGY SYSTEMS

There are three ways in which your body produces energy for your working muscles. We call these the three energy systems. They are the Immediate (or Phosphagen) System, the Anaerobic (or Lactic Acid) System and the Aerobic (or Oxidative) System. The use of these different systems to produce cellular energy (ATP—adenosine tri-phosphate) for your working muscles means that energy is available for all different types of activities, from short bursts such as a fast sprint to longer sustained activity such as a triathlon.

Let's take a glance at each of these systems:

1 *THE IMMEDIATE ENERGY SYSTEM—(ATP-PC)...Up to 10 seconds*

(Primary Activities: sprints, throwing, jumping, power lifting, golf, tennis, basketball)

The Immediate Energy System provides energy at the onset of any exercise and for very short duration, high intensity (95%-100% of maximal effort) activity lasting less than 10 seconds. To produce energy for such high intensity, short duration activity, a high-energy compound called creatine phosphate combines with adenosine diphosphate (ADP) to produce the necessary energy (ATP) required for muscle contraction (McArdle et al. 1999).

Why is it important to know this? If you're doing sprints or intense short duration interval training, you must take into account that muscle energy stores will be completely depleted between 10 seconds and 1 minute and will not be replenished until approximately 2 to 3 minutes after your activity stops. Which means it is most ideal to have a 2 to 3 minute recovery period between sprints.

2 *THE ANAEROBIC ENERGY SYSTEM...Up to 3 minutes*

(Primary Activities: 400M, 800M, Ball Games, weight training, swimming—200M)

This is the primary source of muscle energy (ATP) for maximal "all-out" activity lasting 10 seconds to 3 minutes. For example, during a 2-minute sprint, your body will convert stored muscle sugar (glycogen) into a compound called *pyruvate*. This compound then undergoes a series of chemical reactions in the mitochondria of the cell to assist in the production of ATP for your working muscles. This level of maximal activity cannot be maintained for longer than 3 minutes because your muscles are using energy (ATP) faster than your cells can produce it.

3 ***THE AEROBIC ENERGY SYSTEM...Beyond 3 minutes***
(Primary Activities: walking, jogging, ball games, endurance sports)

The Aerobic System is the body's primary energy source for endurance-type activities lasting longer than 3 minutes. During these activities, sugar stored in your muscles as glycogen, blood glucose, fat and to a lesser degree protein are broken down to produce energy for your working muscles.

▼ WHY IS ALL THIS IMPORTANT?

If you are an athlete or fitness enthusiast, it is essential to understand these systems and how they contribute to the energy production of your particular activity. All three energy systems are important to every activity. However, what varies, is each system's contribution to the production of ATP.

It is also important to note that each of the three energy systems utilizes different nutrients in the production of ATP. The Immediate Energy System uses phospho-creatine (PC), which is stored in the muscle in very limited quantities. Therefore, the effectiveness of this system depends on how well it is trained. A good training program teaches your body to be more effective at replenishing muscle PC stores. This will help to decrease the recovery time between intense short duration activity such as 10 second sprints.

Remember, all these energy systems are very activity specific. Therefore, the PC System can only be trained by doing very high intensity (95%-100% of maximal effort) activity. Examples are: 10 second sprints, jumping, throwing, power-lifting.

On the other hand, the Anaerobic or Lactic Acid Energy System can only use carbohydrates stored in your muscles as glycogen, or blood glucose. To train this system you would do very high intensity work (85%-95% of maximal effort) lasting for 2-3 minutes—sprints, plyometrics, intense weight-training, obstacle course, etc.

The Aerobic System utilizes carbohydrates, fats and protein. To train the body aerobically you would perform moderate to high intensity (75%-85% of maximal effort) activity—jogging, walking, biking, etc. As you can see, what you would eat prior to an activity—or even the day before—will greatly depend on the nature of your activity.

Let's say that your primary activity is basketball, football, or weight-training. In that case, most of your energy would come from stored carbohydrates (glycogen) eaten several hours before your activity. Conversely, if you are a tri-athlete, your body would utilize carbohydrates and fats as your primary energy source and to a lesser degree protein. Keep in mind that fat is used as a primary energy source at low intensities during aerobic activity ONLY. Protein is only used for energy after your carbohydrate stores have been depleted.

HERE'S THE DANGER

IF YOU WORK OUT OR PLAY SPORTS FOR HOURS AT A TIME WITHOUT PROPER NUTRITION, YOUR BODY MAY BREAK DOWN YOUR OWN MUSCLE TISSUE TO USE AS ENERGY. WE CALL THIS MUSCLE CATABOLISM. (BUT IT MIGHT AS WELL BE CALLED MUSCLE CANNIBALISM!)

"Failure is only the opportunity to begin again more intelligently."
—HENRY FORD

ENERGY SYSTEM CONTRIBUTION

ENERGY SYSTEM	Immediate	Lactic Acid	Aerobic
Method of Energy Production:	ANAEROBIC (without oxygen)	ANAEROBIC (without oxygen)	AEROBIC (with oxygen)
Duration:	1-10 seconds	10s to 3 minutes	> 3 minutes
Intensity:	95%-100% (of maximal effort)	85%-95%	<85%
Fuel source:	creatine phosphate	carbohydrates: glycogen,blood glucose	carbohydrates, fats,proteins
Activity:	power lifting throwing, jumping	400m, 800m ball games weight training	endurance sports walking/jogging

Adopted from: Jessica Smith, ME, *Revisiting Energy Systems,* IDEA Source, May 2002.

WHAT SHOULD YOU EAT?

Relative Nutrient Contribution to Exercise at Various Intensities

Nutrient	At Rest	Light to Moderate Intensity	High-Intensity	High-Intensity (Sprints)
PROTEIN	2%-5%	2%-5%	5%-8%	2%
CARBOHYDRATE	35%	40%	70%	95%
FAT	60%	55%	15%	3%

Source: McArdle, W.D., et al 1999. Sports & Exercise Nutrition. New York: Lippincott Williams & Wilkins.

MYTH BUSTER:

I see many people walking on the treadmill for hours every day at very low intensities thinking that they're burning more fat that way. THIS IS NOT THE CASE! While it is true that at lower intensities fat contributes a higher percentage of total calories burned than it does at higher intensities, the *total overall fat calories burned* is greater at higher intensities over an equivalent period of time.

Furthermore, it is important to understand that how much fat your body burns during exercise depends upon your level of cardiovascular fitness and your percentage of lean muscle mass. It is also important to note that after high-intensity training, your metabolism is elevated for several hours. Therefore, the potential for building lean muscle is much greater.

IF YOU'RE AN INTERMEDIATE TO ADVANCE EXERCISER AND YOUR PRIMARY OBJECTIVE IS TO BUILD LEAN MUSCLE TISSUE, I WOULD RECOMMEND INCREASING THE INTENSITY OF YOUR WEIGHT TRAINING AND STICKING TO LOW/MODERATE CARDIOVASCULAR ACTIVITY. YOU WANT TO DO THIS, BECAUSE TO BUILD LEAN MUSCLE, YOU NEED TO CONSUME A TREMENDOUS AMOUNT OF PROTEIN AND CARBOHYDRATES. AND HIGH INTENSITY CARDIOVASCULAR TRAINING BURNS A LOT OF CARBOHYDRATES.

THE NUTRIENT MAKE-UP OF FOOD

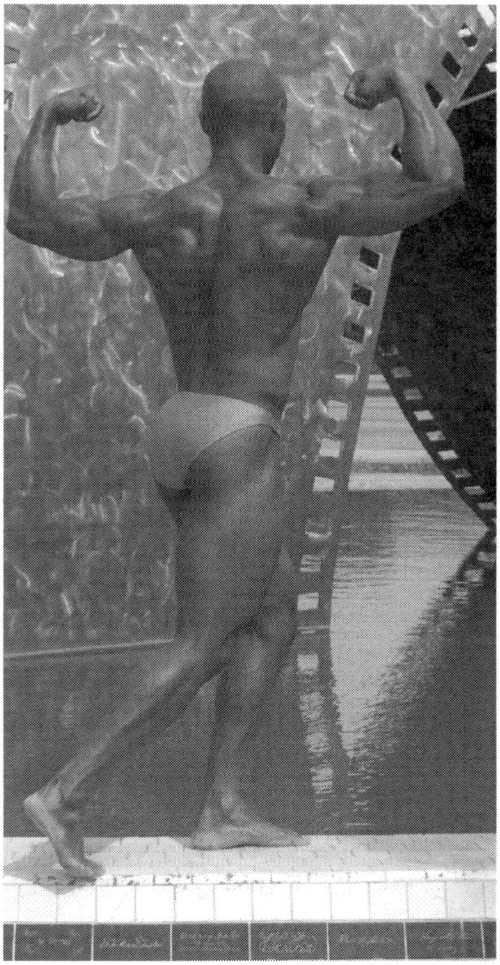

▼ PROTEIN

Protein is one of the 2 most important nutrients you'll need to build muscle; water is the other. Without adequate protein consumption, you simply will not change the look of your body because you're not going to grow muscle.

Collagen, catabolism/anabolism cycle

Remember, your body is constructed of protein. The amino acids in the foods you eat are the only available source of protein available to your body to facilitate growth of skin, hair, nails, bones, teeth, etc. Furthermore, protein helps to form collagens which create cartilage, ligaments and tendons. Collagens also help to strengthen the cell walls of veins and arteries. During exercise, your muscle tissue is being broken down in a process called catabolism. Without adequate protein intake your body will be in a perpetual state of catabolism. Adequate protein intake helps the body to complete the catabolism/anabolism cycle. During the anabolism cycle, your body actually builds new lean muscle tissue.

Non-essential/Essential Amino Acids

Protein is made up of amino acids. There are two types of amino acids: non-essential (dispensable) and essential (indispensable). Your body is capable of synthesizing non-essential amino acids on its own. However, there are eight essential amino acids that your body cannot produce. These are found in animal protein in the right balance—meat, fish, eggs, poultry, etc.

Vegetarians take note: Keep in mind that plant sources of protein are very low in one or more indispensable amino acids. If you are a vegetarian, *proper food combining* is essential to get all the necessary essential amino acids your body needs.

Here's a cute little saying that contains a simple food combining formula:

My **G**randmother **L**ikes **N**uts and **S**eeds

M = milk or dairy products
G = grains
L = legumes—beans, peas, etc.
N = nuts
S = seeds

The combination of any two of the above food groups will give you a complete amino acid profile or a complete protein. For example, Grains & Legumes (rice and beans) is a complete protein.

▼ CARBOHYDRATES

Not all carbs are created equal...

Carbohydrates give you energy to train hard and to perform your other daily activities. Your brain also needs carbohydrates to function. Are all carbohydrates basically the same? You sugar addicts wish they were. Carbohydrates can be classified into two groups: simple sugar—found in candies, fruit, fruit juices, syrups and processed foods—and complex carbohydrates—found in whole grains, vegetables, beans, etc.

For all you sugar babies, I know it's the shame
But not all carbs are the same
You've got candy and cookies and the whole dessert game
These carbs are just gonna add pounds to your frame
But the other carbs - like oatmeal, my favorite
-now that's a different game...

It is important to note that the body treats simple sugars quite differently than it does complex carbohydrates. Yes, they are both broken down into glucose, but due to the significant difference in their molecular structure they are handled very differently.

Simple sugars

Simple sugars are what we call monosaccharides or disaccharides. This simply means that they are constructed of either one (mono) or two (di) molecules of sugar (saccharide). Glucose is a monosaccharide, so is fructose, the sugar found in fruit and fruit juices. Sucrose or table sugar is a disaccharide. It is composed of glucose and fructose, which makes it the sweetest of them all. Lactose is another disaccharide found in milk. It is made up of glucose and galactose.

Simple sugars are released very quickly into the bloodstream. Your pancreas responds just as quickly by secreting insulin into the bloodstream. Insulin is like a fat jailer. This notorious hormone is responsible for facilitating the removal of excess sugar from your bloodstream and putting it into fat cells. Insulin also prevents the opposing hormone glucagon—which is responsible for unlocking your fat stores—from entering the bloodstream. The result is that simple sugars are more easily converted to body fat. This also happens when you eat simple sugars and fats together at the same meal, in the case of fast foods.

Don't be fooled by foods at your local health food store that are sweetened with fruit juice. They are still simple sugars, because they contain fructose which is just as easily metabolized into triglycerides, a fat. From a sugar standpoint, a glass of orange juice is no different than a can of regular cola. Therefore, my recommendation is to eat your fruit and drink water. This way you're ingesting far less simple sugars. This doesn't apply to competitive athletes (you should be drinking a beverage containing simple carbohydrates during your game or match). However, if you're trying to lose fat, I recommend eating only green apples, green pears and berries for the first month of your transformation program. (If you can coordinate your program to coincide with St. Patrick's Day, the green becomes less of an issue.)

▼ FATS

Fat serves a vital purpose in your body. Fat protects your organs and provides fat-soluble vitamins and is also necessary for hormonal production. At least 15-20% of your daily calories should come from good fats (unsaturated) such as avocado, extra virgin olive oil, canola oil and flax seed oil.

▼ CARBOHYDRATES, PROTEINS & FATS

How do these nutrients contribute to muscle energy production (ATP)?

CARBOHYDRATES in the form of glucose are used to produce ATP while the Aerobic and Anaerobic (Lactic Acid) Energy Systems are in use (sprints, 400M, 800M, ball games, jogging, walking, etc).

PROTEINS — During exercise, proteins in the form of amino acids contribute very little to ATP production (less than 5%). However, metabolism of amino acids can contribute up to 20% of muscle energy production under extreme conditions, such as starvation or after several hours of prolonged exercise.

FATS — At rest and during low intensity activity, fats—in the form of fatty acids—can be used to produce ATP (muscle energy) aerobically only…that is, only during endurance activity lasting longer than 3 minutes.

Why is all this important for an athlete or avid exerciser to know? Two simple reasons:

(1) If you do not consume the right types of foods several hours prior to your activity, you may end up stressing the body too much to compensate for your lack of energy, therefore, poor performance.

(2) If you exercise while your body is in starvation mode (constantly skipping meals over long periods of time), your own muscle tissue, which is 22% protein, will be broken down to provide energy for your activity. THIS IS NOT A GOOD THING!!

EATING TO BURN FAT, BUILD MUSCLE AND ENHANCE YOUR ATHLETIC PERFORMANCE:

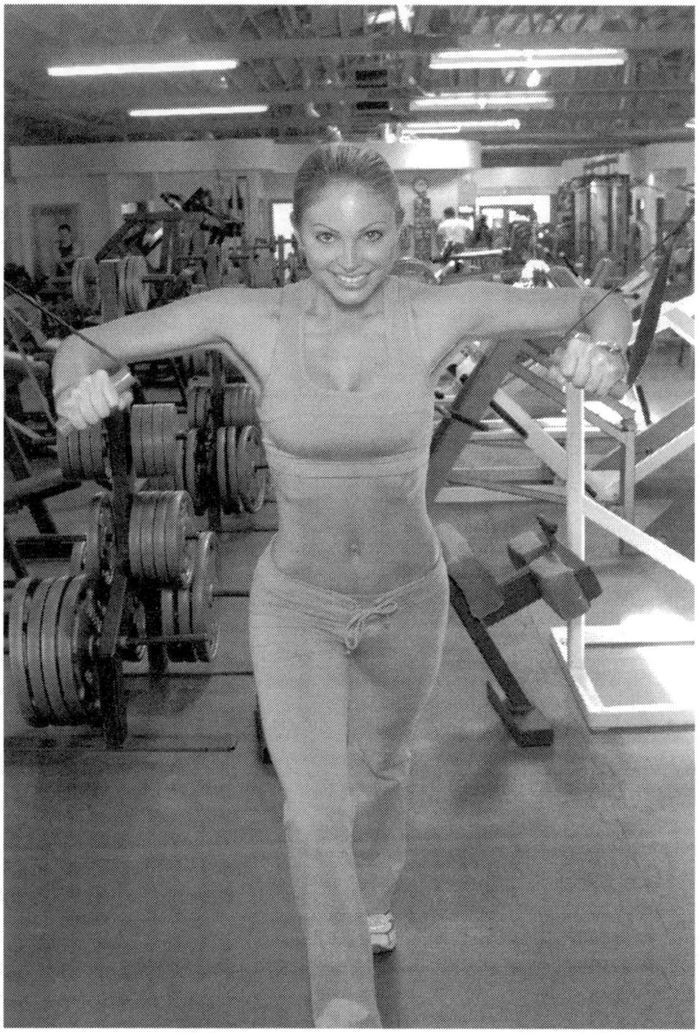

▼ FAT BURNING

To maximize fat burning, do your cardiovascular exercise first thing in the morning on an empty stomach or in the evening 3 hours after your mid-afternoon meal. Another great time to do cardio is right after a really intense weight training session lasting 45 – 60 minutes. After such an intense weight training session, your glycogen stores (the body's main energy source) will have been significantly depleted, therefore your system is forced to switch to fat and protein for energy.

The problem with doing intense training for longer than one hour is this . . . your glycogen stores are significantly depleted and the body can only metabolize fat aerobically. Therefore, if you continue to do intense weight training work for more than about 1 hour, your body will start breaking down protein to get the necessary energy for you to continue training. This is counter-productive if your objective is to develop lean muscle mass. And I'm assuming it is, otherwise, why would you be doing weight training?

Fat Burning Supplements:

"All you have to do is take
one No Mo Flab tablet in the morning
and you can eat absolutely anything you want
and YOU WON'T GET FAT!
That's a guarantee!
For a limited time a one-month supply
(normally worth hundreds of dollars)
is just $69.95.
Act now and say goodbye to fat forever!"

Way too close to too many infomercials as it is . . .

Like diets, there are hundreds of so-called "fat burners" on the market. Obviously the vast majority add up to nothing more than marketing hype. The only supplements I recommend for fat burning are *JuicePlus+® Thins,* a fruit and vegetable concentrate in capsule form, Essential Fatty acids and a good *protein powder.* The Thins contain fiber from a tropical Asian fruit, Garcinia Cambogia, which naturally increases the effectiveness of insulin and promotes oxidation of fatty acids. A study published in *The Journal of the American Nutraceutical Association* found that a combination of the JuicePlus+® Thins, JuicePlus+® Capsules (fruit and vegetable concentrate) and the JuicePlus+® Complete meal replacement, helped participants to lose more fat weight and increased their lean muscle mass after only 60 days.

POPULAR "FAT BURNING" SUPPLEMENTS REVIEWED

L-CARNITINE

What is it?

Carnitine is a non-essential amino acid that the body synthesizes from another amino acid, Lysine. Red meat is also a good dietary source. While Carnitine has many functions in the body, it is best known for transferring fatty acids—In the body, fats break down to fatty acids— across cell membranes to the mitochondria where they can be burned (oxidized) as energy.

What is it supposed to do?

Carnitine is sold primarily as a sports supplement. The theory is that additional Carnitine will help to shuttle more fatty acids across cell membranes to be burned as energy rather than stored as body fat.

What does the research say?

Clinical studies on the effects of Carnitine on exercise performance and metabolism during exercise have been conflicting and at most very unimpressive.

Recommendation:

Although Carnitine has many potential health benefits for people with certain medical conditions, it hasn't been shown to be effective as a weight loss supplement. The bottom line is, it is very expensive and is probably a waste of your money.

CHROMIUM

What is it?

Chromium is a mineral that acts as a coenzyme to insulin, the fat storage hormone. It assists in regulating blood sugar and fat metabolism.

What is it supposed to do?

The presumption here is that anything that helps to regulate blood sugar and fat metabolism will also help with food cravings and weight loss.

What does the research say?

Again, like Carnitine, the research on Chromium is conflicting. One study shows that it is effective in the fat-loss process, and another shows that it has no effect.

Recommendation:

The truth is I have never met anyone who lost any weight just by adding Chromium to his/her diet. Therefore, as a fat-loss supplement you could probably do without it. On the other hand, it is well documented that a large portion of the American population is deficient in Chromium, since it is stripped away in the processing of most processed foods. For this reason, supplementing with 300-500 mcg/day could be beneficial.

EPHEDRINE/CAFFEINE

What is it?

The thermogenic products most popular among the weight-loss and bodybuilding arenas are combinations of ephedrine and caffeine. Ephedrine is a drug derived from the herb Ephedra or MaHuang. It is a bronchodilator used in asthma medication, opening the air passageway leading to and from the lungs. Ephedrine is also a natural appetite suppressant. Caffeine, on the other hand, is extracted from Guarana, Kola Nut or Green Tea. As I mentioned before, both ephedrine and caffeine are stimulants. They are also diuretics, meaning they excrete water from the body.

What is it supposed to do?

Ephedrine and caffeine are what we call thermogenics because they can increase the rate at which thermogenisis (the production of heat) occurs in the body, thereby, increasing metabolic rate.

What does the research say?

The research is very conclusive, together, ephedrine and caffeine is a very effective fat-loss compound.

Recommendation:

Let's face it, every drug has side effects and contraindications. The primary concern that I have with thermogenics is that the vast majority of people who are lured into using them are either overweight or obese. They also tend to suffer from hypertension, thyroid or cardiorespiratory issues. These are the people for whom ephedrine and caffeine are contraindicated or strongly not advised. If you have any of the above conditions, you do not want to be on stimulants because you could have a stroke or die.

If you are a competitive athlete, this compound may be helpful in your fat-loss efforts. However, I would not recommend using it without the assistance of a trained professional. The majority of studies I have looked at used 20 mg of ephedrine and 200 mg of caffeine three times per day. Keep in mind that both ephedrine and caffeine are addictive substances and should not be used for longer than 4-5 weeks at a time. If you use them, I would strongly suggest doing so for only 4-5 weeks, then taking an 8-10 week recovery period. More frequent usage may compromise your body's natural adrenal production. Would I personally recommend them to a client? The answer is emphatically NO!

FAT BLOCKERS

What are they?

Xenical is a drug and Chitosan (which is extracted from shellfish) is a supplement that blocks the absorption of fat in the digestive track.

What are they supposed to do?

Both these products attract fat molecules and rap them up into big "fat balls" making it impossible for your body to absorb them.

Recommendation:

Stay away from these products! Whenever you block the absorption of fats you also block the absorption of essential vitamins, A, D, E and K...these are fat soluble vitamins. More importantly, however, is the fact that you will also block the absorption of *essential fatty acids* that are critical to almost every function in your body. These are called *essential* because your body cannot make them; they must be supplied through your diet. Some side effects include oily discharge, anal leakage, intestinal cramping, gas with discharge, diarrhea, loose and oily stools, and the list goes on.

DHEA

What is it?

Dehydroepiandrosterone (DHEA) is a steroid hormone produced in the adrenal glands. It is called "The Mother of All Hormones." It is the hormone from which all sex hormones, estrogen and testosterone are created.

What is it supposed to do?

DHEA is marketed as a cure-all for almost every ailment you can think of—weight loss, immune system, heart disease and many more.

What does the research say?

The research is very impressive when it comes to immune enhancement, anti-cancer benefits and even cognitive functioning. However, as a weight loss supplement, DHEA has only been able to make mice lose weight.

Recommendations:

There are many positive benefits to DHEA supplementation in people over forty with reduced DHEA levels. However, only a blood test can tell you if your DHEA levels are reduced in comparison to others in your age group. Generally, only about 25-100mg per day is needed to have a positive effect on lean mass and bone density in older adults. You should only take DHEA supplementation if your levels are low and your doctor prescribes it. Otherwise, don't mess around with your hormones, because they are all inter-related, and you may suffer unwanted consequences.

ESSENTIAL FATTY ACIDS

What are they?

Essential Fatty Acids (EFA's) are two types of unsaturated fats that cannot be made by the body and are vitally necessary for thousands of biochemical processes in the body to take place. These are linoleic acid (omega-6 fatty acid) and linolenic acid (omega-3 fatty acid).

What are they supposed to do?

EFA's play an enormous role in the body, including the production of steroid hormones that regulate the production of testosterone.

What does the research say?

The research clearly shows that people on very low-fat diets (which of course would be low in EFA's) experience a significant decrease in testosterone production. This is bad news if you're trying to build muscle or lose body fat.

Recommendation:

Add some cold water fish such as salmon, trout or mackerel to your diet at least a couple times per week. Flaxseed oil, Soybean oil and canola oil are also good sources of EFA's. Try to add a teaspoon of one of these oils to your meals. Another option is to use EFA supplements. This is one fat that definitely will not make you fat. And will help to increase your HDL (good) cholesterol and accelerate fat loss.

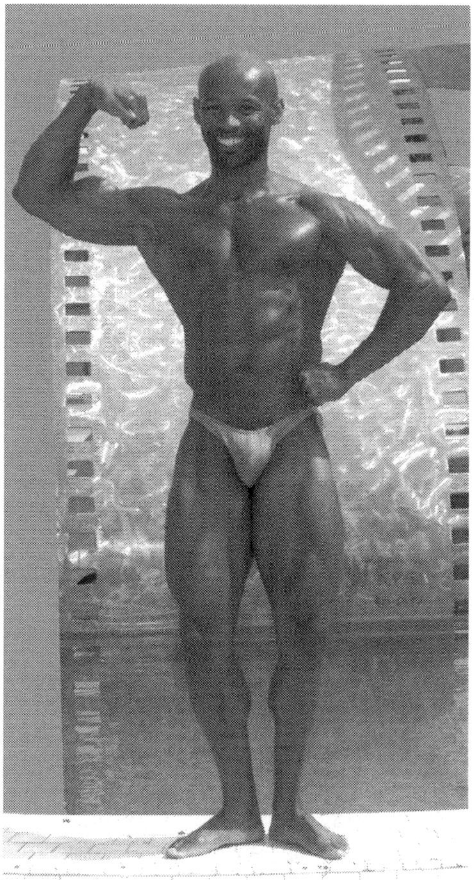

▼ BUILDING LEAN MUSCLE

To build lean muscle you've got to eat early, eat late and eat often! Last year I was able to put on 10 pounds of solid lean muscle, naturally, in just 6 months. How did I do it? By having a meal every 2 to 3 hours and doing what I call "bone-crushing" weight training 4 to 5 times a week. The "experts" will tell you that this is impossible. They'll say that it is mostly water and fat. You be the judge. Take a look at my pictures. I was pretty well dehydrated for my show and I don't see any fat anywhere. Incidentally, I took first place in my weight class at that show.

Remember, weight training requires lots of complex carbohydrates. That's where you get the energy to train hard. Also keep in mind that it is most beneficial to drink a simple carbohydrate beverage immediately after your training to replenish your glycogen stores. Research shows that a post-workout mixture of simple sugar, creatine and glutamine is best.

SUPPLEMENTS FOR BUILDING AND MAINTAINING LEAN MUSCLE

When it comes to supplements, the truth of the matter is we don't know if there are any side effects from long term use of creatine, glutamine, HMB and CLA. However, current research shows that they are effective in helping you build and maintain lean muscle tissue. However, *they will only work for you if you're doing very intense weight training.* They have not been shown to be effective in endurance training. You decide whether or not to use them and please consult with your physician. I use them for 4 to 6 weeks at a time then I take a 6 to 8 week break. I also use the JuicePlus+® Capsules (fruit and vegetable concentrate) 3 to 4 times a day, in addition to EFA's—Essential Fatty Acids.

CREATINE

What is it?

Creatine (methylguanido-acetic acid) is a natural compound synthesized in your body from the amino acids arginine, methionine and glycine. It is produced in the liver and transported in the blood where it is taken up by working muscle cells. It is then converted to creatine phosphate (CP) or "phosphocreatine."

What is it supposed to do?

As you may recall from our discussion of the three energy systems, phosphocreatine is used to produced ATP (adenosine triphosphate) at the onset of any exercise and for very short duration, high-intensity (95%-100% of maximal effort) activity lasting less than 10 seconds. In addition, creatine helps to build lean muscle mass and speeds up recovery.

What does the research say?

There is a wealth of research data showing the effectiveness of creatine in building lean muscle mass. Simply put, the stuff makes you work a lot harder in the gym.

Recommendation:

The best times to use creatine monohydrate is before and right after your workout. There is a recommended 1week "loading" phase of 30 grams/day, however, I have never found this to be necessary. 5-10 grams/day is quite sufficient for a 4-5 week period. Again, these supplements haven't been on the market long enough for us to have any concrete long term studies done. However, we do know that supplementing with creatine does shut down your body's natural creatine production. Therefore, I always recommend taking a 6-8 week recovery period. Personally, I don't want to shut down any of my body's natural processes for long periods of time.

GLUTAMINE

What is it?

Glutamine is an amino acid that the body synthesizes from other amino acids, namely glutamic acid, valine and isoleucine. It is required for proper functioning of your immune system, pancreas, kidneys and liver. Glutamine is also an important building block for the most powerful antioxidant in the body—glutathione.

What is it supposed to do?

Your body uses very large quantities of glutamine everyday to maintain the above mentioned systems. However, when more is needed than is produced or taken in through your diet (for example, while under extreme stress such as exercise), muscle tissue is robbed of its stored glutamine. This is considered a catabolic or muscle wasting process.

What does the research say?

Studies show that glutamine supplementation can have anti-catabolic effects. That is, it helps to preserve muscle tissue.

Recommendation:

Use 2-3 grams of glutamine after your workouts and before going to bed. I mix it in water or put it in my meal replacement shakes.

HMB

What is it?

HMB (beta-hydroxy beta-methylbutyrate) is produced in the body from the amino acid leucine. It can also be found in grapefruit and catfish.

What is it supposed to do?

HMB is believed to minimize the breakdown of muscle tissue and may even double the muscle-building and fat-burning effects of exercise.

What does the research say?

The research on HMB is quite extensive. One study published in the *Journal of Applied Physiology* revealed that athletes who supplemented with 3 grams of HMB per day gain 3 times as much lean muscle mass as the placebo group.

Recommendation:

Supplementing with 2-3 grams of HMB per day may prove to be beneficial in your muscle-building quest over time.

CLA

What is it?

Conjugated Lenoleic Acid (CLA) is a fatty acid that is derived from the essential fatty acid lenoleic acid (omega-6 fatty acid). It is found in meats and dairy products. It has also been shown to affect the metabolism of animals.

What is it supposed to do?

CLA is believed to reduce body fat and increase lean muscle mass.

What does the research say?

The animal studies on CLA are very impressive. However, the human studies are conflicting and inconclusive.

Recommendation:

CLA has excellent health benefits such as anti-oxidant and anti-cancer properties. At present, we cannot say with certainty that it does enhance the fat-loss process and increase lean muscle mass. However, it is a very safe product and might be worth your while, if you feel like experimenting and you've got the money to do so. Most of the human studies used 3-5 grams per day, which is quite expensive.

TESTOSTERONE PRECURSOR

What is it?

Androstene is a precursor hormone between DHEA and testosterone that aids the liver in synthesizing other steroid hormones.

What is it supposed to do?

According to the ads, it is supposed to give you the strength of Hercules and enough sexual stamina to outlast the best adult film stars.

What does the research say?

There is little scientific evidence to support the claims about Androstene's anabolic muscle-building effectiveness.

Recommendation:

It is never a good idea to mess around with your hormones. Remember, whenever you mess with one, it always affects the others—they are all inter-related. The body has its own mechanism for balancing testosterone and estrogen. Therefore, it is irrational to think that you can increase your testosterone levels without a significant estrogen response. Stay away from these drugs or you may find yourself bald, aggressive, moody and worst of all, visiting your doctor or surfing the net for Viagra prescriptions.

Researchers at George Washington University found that people who have been successful in transforming their bodies all had an "emotional trigger" that helps to clarify their reasons for wanting to change their bodies in the first place. What's your big WHY?

A study published in the New England Journal of Medicine found that women who use estrogen replacement therapy have a 50% chance of developing ovarian cancer.

▼ ENDURANCE ATHLETES

If you are an endurance athlete, it is a good practice to regularly ingest some form of simple sugar and electrolyte mixture. It is especially important to keep replenishing your electrolytes if you're training or competing for several hours at a time.

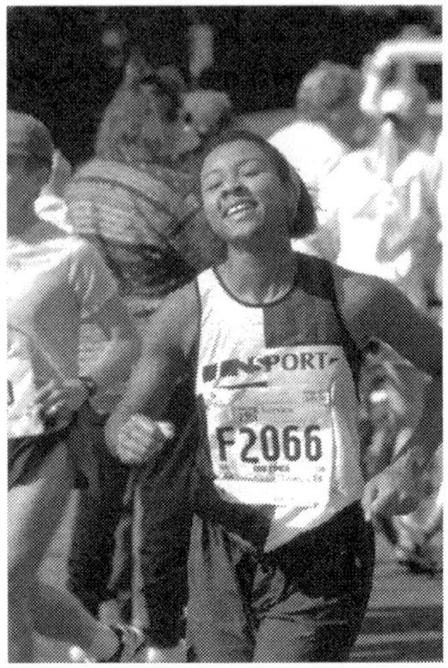

Drinking water alone while you're sweating for several hours may lead to hyponatremia — sometimes called water intoxication. This can happen when levels of sodium, or other electrolytes (potassium, calcium and bicarbonate), in the blood drop to dangerously low levels. When the concentration of electrolytes in the blood gets too low compared to the amount inside the cells — either because you drank too much water, took in too little electrolytes, or both — water rushes into the cells. The result is dangerous swelling — particularly in the brain — that can lead to brain damage, coma and death.

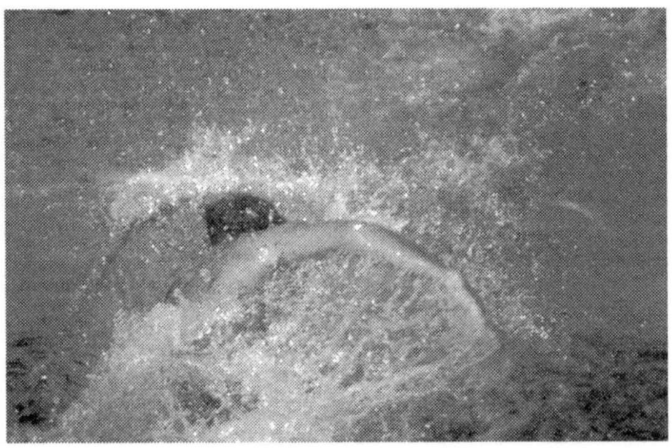

Endurance athletes need to know that the two most important sources of energy are carbohydrates — simple and complex — and fats. Remember that it takes several hours for the body to completely digest complex carbohydrates and fats. Therefore, you should always be thinking ahead. Your energy for a morning practice or competition will come from what you ate the previous evening. Similarly, your energy for an afternoon practice or competition will come largely from what you ate in the morning. In addition, a whole food concentrate in capsule form will give your body the necessary nutrients it needs to perform efficiently.

> **"Is there life before death?"**
>
> —Belfast Graffito

Don't forget: PERFORMANCE EQUALS NUTRITION!

One of my dearest clients is a little 9-year-old aspiring professional tennis player. She has great natural abilities and excellent coaching, but before I started working with her she never gave 100% during her practices or matches because her eating habits were simply terrible. The first week I worked with her I noticed that she would tire quickly, and how could she not, she had already played two hours of tennis. My first question to her was, "What did you have to eat today?" Her response, "Two hot dogs."

I promptly ended our session, sent her inside to eat and proceeded to give her mother a nutrition lecture for the next hour. Remember, PERFORMANCE EQUALS NUTRITION!

To work a body is quite sublime
to waste that body should be crime
I'm smart enough to realize
that I should try to exercise
But I really don't have the time.

— COUCH POTATO LIMERICK

IMPORTANT POINTS TO REMEMBER

1 Diet is extremely important to energy metabolism and exercise performance.

2 Muscle glycogen stores (stored carbohydrates) can be depleted in as little as 40 minutes of intense prolonged exercise, such as distance running or intense weight training.

3 Sports in which glycogen depletion may occur include: football, soccer, basketball, tennis, triathlon, extended periods of weight training.

4 24-48 hours is required to fully restore muscle glycogen levels...provided adequate dietary carbohydrates are consumed.

5 Low carbohydrate diets result in low muscle glycogen stores and poor exercise performance.

6 Research suggests that consumption of foods with a moderate to high glycemic index in the 24 hours after high intensity training or during competition extending for several days is preferable for replenishing muscle glycogen stores. *Burke, Collier & Hergreaus,* 1993—*Journal of Applied Physiology,* 75,1019-23

7 Your body builds and repairs muscle tissue while you are sleeping. Furthermore, 90% of the growth hormone necessary to build and repair muscle tissue is secreted during the first 4 hours of deep sleep.

8 To build lean muscle mass, drink at least 1 gallon of water daily. Remember, muscle is 78% water.

HOW MANY CALORIES SHOULD YOU EAT?

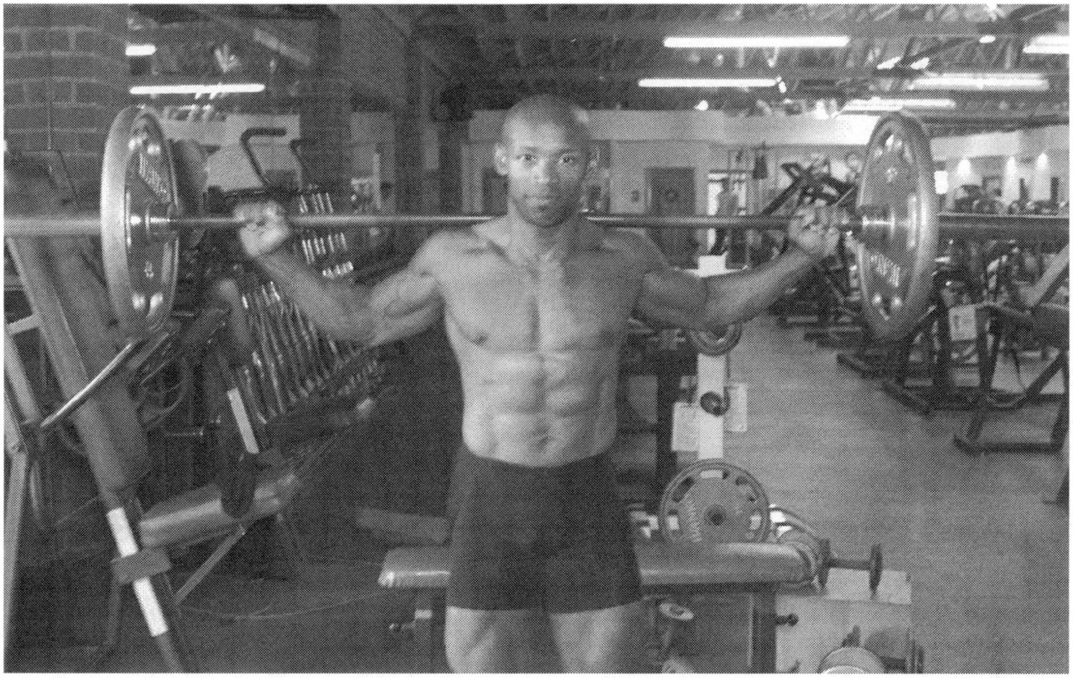

The amount of calories you will need daily will depend on several factors: your age, weight, height, percent body fat and of course your fitness goals.

▼ BMR (Basal Metabolic Rate)

First things first: let's talk about the minimum amount of calories your body needs daily just to keep you alive. We call this your BMR or Basal Metabolic Rate. That's the amount of calories your body needs for respiration, circulation, to keep your heart beating, your lungs, liver and other vital organs functioning.

CALCULATING YOUR BMR

The easiest way to calculate your BMR is simply to add a zero to your weight. For example, a woman who weighs 140 lbs. requires 1400 calories just to keep the body's vital organs functioning...add a zero to 140. A man who weighs 170 lbs.. requires at least 1700 calories daily.

NEVER EAT FEWER CALORIES THAN YOUR BMR. IF YOU DO, YOUR BODY WILL START TO FEED ON ITSELF!!! A VERY UGLY EXPERIENCE...

THE HARRIS-BENEDICT EQUATION
(BMR based on total body weight)

MEN: BMR = 66 + (13.7 X wt in kg) + (5 X ht in cm)
– (6.8 X age in years)

WOMEN: BMR = 655 + (9.6 X wt. in kg) + (1.8 X ht in cm)
– (4.7 X age in years)

Note: 1 inch = 2.54 cm / 1 Kilogram = 2.2 lbs.

EXAMPLE:
You are a female
You are 35 years old
You are 5′5″ tall (65 inches = 165.1 cm)
You weigh 140 lbs.. (63.6 kg)
Your BMR = 655 + (9.6 X 63.6) + (1.8 X 165.1) – (4.7 X 35)
= 1405 calories/day

Oh but Dr. Del, I know me. I'll never count calories...

Take heart, this information is primarily for those of you who need to accurately calculate your daily caloric needs. If you're not interested in doing these calculations (or just plain won't or maybe never got higher than a D+ in math) I'll show you an easier way when we get to your meal plan.

"Freedom of will is the ability to do gladly that which I must do."
— CARL JUNG

▼ YOUR TOTAL DAILY CALORIES:

Now that you know your BMR, you can calculate your total amount of calories your body burns each day. We call this your **Total Daily Energy Expenditure (TDEE).**

TDEE = BMR x Activity Index

Example:
Your BMR is 1405
Your Activity Index is 1.8
Your TDEE = 1405 X 1.8 = 2,529 calories

ACTIVITY INDEX

Average Couch Potato	= BMR X 1.2	Sedentary
Light activity	= BMR X 1.4	Light exercise 1-3 days/week
Moderately active	= BMR X 1.6	Moderate exercise 3-5 days/week
Very active	= BMR X 1.8	Hard exercise 6-7 days/week
Intense activity	= BMR X 2.0	Intense workouts or very physical job
Extended intense activity	= BMR X 2.5	Extremely high intensity, high duration sports

A SIMPLER WAY OF CALCULATING YOUR BMR IS BASED ON YOUR LEAN BODY MASS.

KATCH-MCARDLE FORMULA
BMR (Men & Women) = 370 + (21.6 x lean mass in kg)
TDEE = BMR X Activity level

This is a more accurate equation if you are either very muscular or very obese. Remember, TDEE is your maintenance level—the daily amount of calories required to maintain your current weight.

<u>TO LOSE FAT WEIGHT</u>

Reduce Daily Calories (TDEE) by 15-20% = Calorie deficit

Example:
Your weight is 140 lbs..
Your TDEE is 2000 calories.
Your Calorie deficit is 20% of TDEE = 400 calories.
Your Optimal Calorie intake for weight loss = 1600 calories.

<u>TO GAIN LEAN BODY WEIGHT</u>

Increase Daily Caloric intake (TDEE) by 15-20%

Example:
Your weight is 140 lbs..
Your TDEE is 2000.
Your Optimal Caloric intake for weight gain = 2000 + (300-400)
= 2300-2400 calories.

HOW MANY CALORIES SHOULD YOU EAT?

1 gm. protein = 4 calories
1 gm. fat = 9 calories
1 gm. carbohydrate = 4 calories
1 ounce = 28 gm.

Example:
You're interested in fat loss.
Your weight is 140 lbs..
Your TDEE is 2000 calories.

Your Calorie deficit is 20% of TDEE = 400 calories
Your Optimal Calorie intake for weight loss = 1600 calories = TDEE (Optimal)

Protein = 30% = .30 X TDEE (Optimal) = 480 cal. divide by 4 = 120 gms/day
Carbohydrates = 50% = .50 X TDEE (Optimal) = 800 cal. divide by 4 = 200 gms/day
Fat = 20% = .20 X TDEE (Optimal) = 500 cal. divide by 9 = 56 gms/day

Again, keep in mind: the types of carbohydrates I recommend that you eat are very low in calories and very dense in nutrition. Therefore, the percentage is low but the amount of food you're actually eating is a lot.

▼ RATIO OF PROTEIN, CARBOHYDRATES AND FATS

Macro-nutrient ratios are still being debated by the "experts". The amount you need is based on several factors: your body's ability to metabolize those nutrients, your activity level and your goals.

MY PHILOSOPHY

Always eat to build lean muscle and lose body fat!

This requires more protein and water than is needed by the average non-active individual. When it comes to carbohydrates, I recommend eating fibrous vegetables, yams, legumes, oats, brown and wild rice. These contain far less calories than the more highly processed foods like pasta, breads and other baked goods. Since these foods are lower in calories your total daily caloric percentage will also be lower, yet you'll be eating more food.

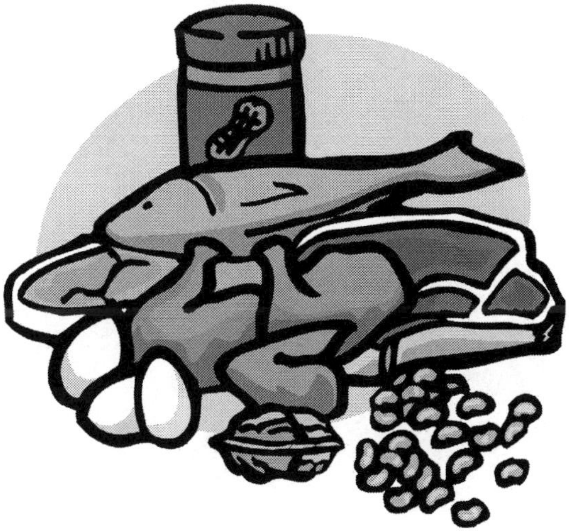

Plenty of protein, gallons of H_2O

You'll build that muscle and watch the love handles go

If you don't begin, you'll never know

Give it a try...so I can say "I told you so"

Start it now, so you can say "Del told me so."

My recommendation: **KEEP IT SIMPLE!**

Goal:	Fat Loss	Weight Gain (lean mass)	Endurance Athlete
Protein	30-40%	30-40%	15-20%
Carbohydrates	40-50%	50-60%	60-70%
Fat	15-20%	10-20%	20-30%

DON'T FORGET: YOU'VE GOT TO EAT FAT TO LOSE FAT!

Be you diplomat or acrobat, hot mama or cool cat
Republican or Democrat
This is where it's at:
You've gotta eat fat to lose fat
Don't you ever forget that:
You've gotta eat fat to lose fat

Studies on Glucosamine indicate
a 50 - 70 percent reduction
in joint pain symptoms
after only 6 to 8 weeks.
Some Researchers say that
Glucosamine may also help to
maintain and rebuild joint cartilage.

KIDS & NUTRITION

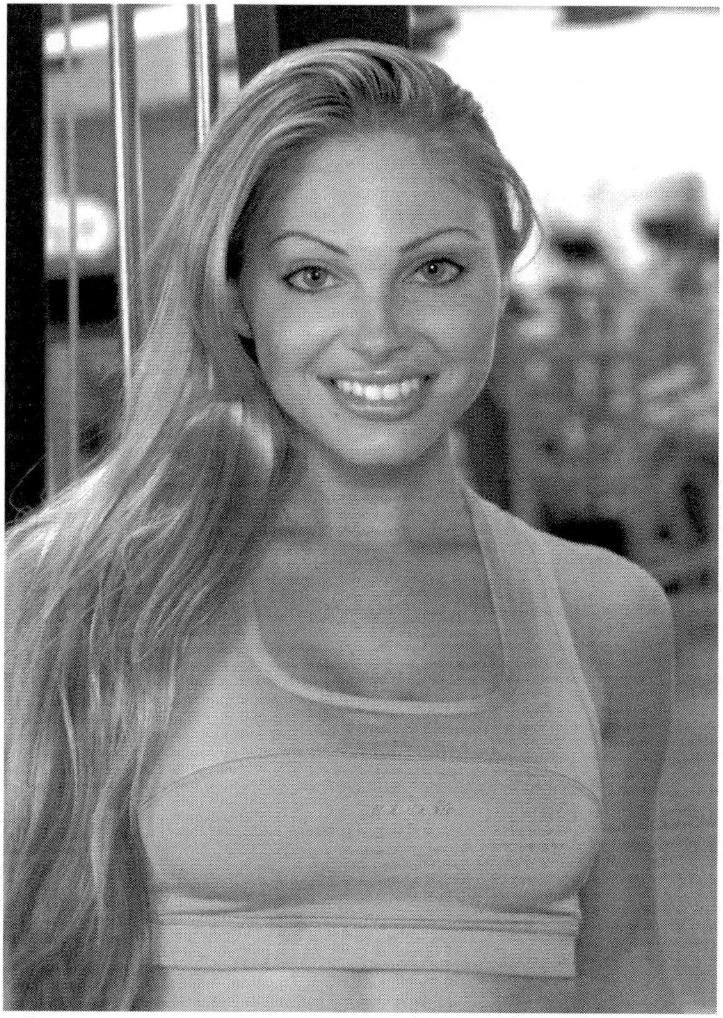

▼ FEEDING OUR FUTURE SUPERSTARS

America is at war over the nutritional health of our children. Unfortunately, we're miserably losing that war. Parents are "too busy" to make sure their children eat balanced nutritious meals. Even more to the point, most parents don't have a clue what "eating right" means. As a result, our children turn to TV commercials to give them their nutritional education. This is not good!

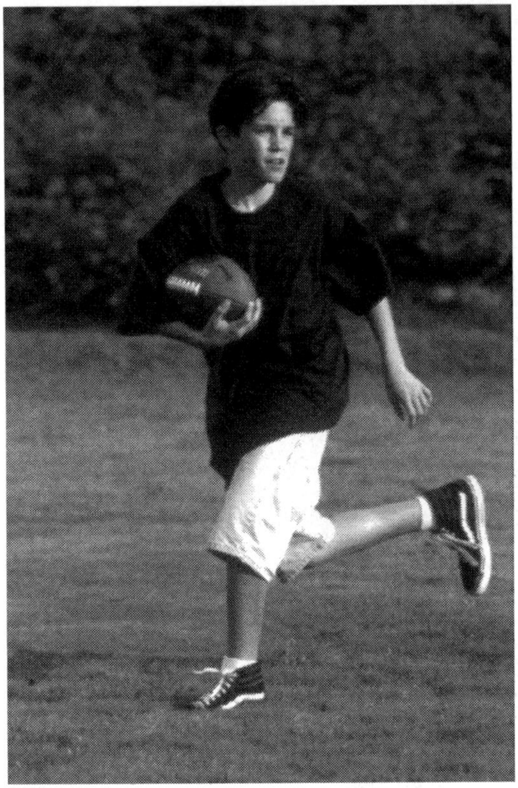

God bless Ronald McDonald, but you don't want him teaching your kids nutrition.

The statistics below clearly demonstrate the negative impact that the multi-billion dollar junk food and fast food industries are having on the health of our children:

- 1 in 4 children in the US today is seriously overweight
- 40 million American children have abnormally high cholesterol levels.
- By age 12, 70% of children have the beginning stages of hardening of the arteries.
- Over the last 20 years the number of extremely overweight children has nearly doubled, and the number of overweight children has increased by more than 50%.

WHAT CAN WE DO ABOUT THIS?

The answer is clear. We must encourage our kids to eat more fresh raw fruits and vegetables, high quality protein, complex carbohydrates, such as whole wheat breads, cereals low in sugar and high in fiber—at least 3 grams, and my personal favorite: oatmeal. And we have to break out of our fast food comas. We must limit the amounts of processed and fast foods they eat to at most once per week. Most importantly, we must lead by example.

> "When we truly care for ourselves, it becomes possible to care far more profoundly about other people."
>
> — Edna LeShan

MODEL GOOD EATING HABITS AND YOUR CHILDREN WILL FOLLOW!

My dad calls my mom "Blimpie."

She calls him "Fatty."

They taught me how to eat.

When I grow up, will I look like mommy and daddy?

As parents, it's important to be proactive about your child's nutritional habits. In addition to becoming more aware of what they're putting in their bodies, you can join forces with one of the many nutrition foundations whose primary objective is to educate families about the importance of good nutrition.

One such organization is the JuicePlus+® *Children's Research Foundation* (JPCRF). JPCRF has a *Children's Health Study* designed to determine what effect adding a whole food fruit and vegetable concentrate (like JuicePlus+®) to the family diet can have on children's health and learning ability. To encourage families to participate, the foundation is providing each child with free JuicePlus+®.

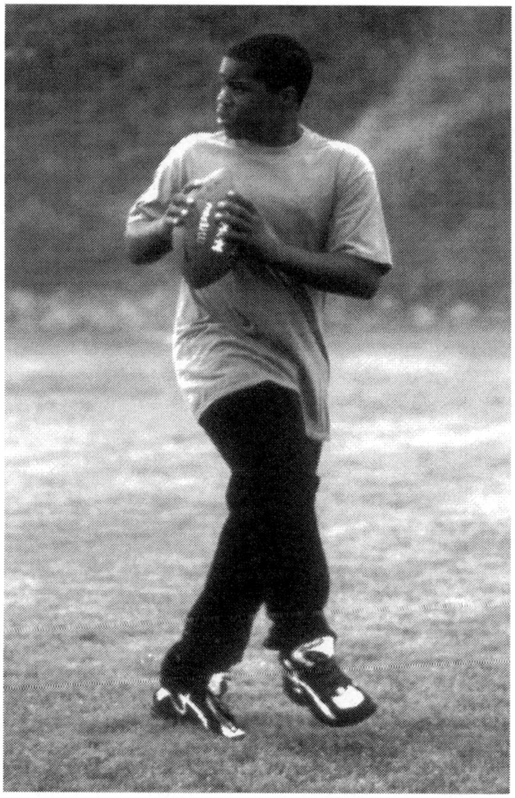

To learn more about the *Children's Health Study,* visit my website at http://www.delmillers.com and click on my children's nutrition page.

"The flowers of all the tomorrows are planted in the seeds of today."
— Ancient Chinese Proverb

▼ WHAT SHOULD YOUR CHILD BE EATING?

- 6-11 servings daily of complex carbohydrates rich in vitamins, minerals and fiber – wheat, rice, oats, millet, corn, whole wheat bread, pasta.
- 6-10 servings daily of fresh fruits and vegetables of a variety of colors – tomatoes, spinach, broccoli, carrots, sweet potatoes, squash, peaches, bananas, apples and oranges.
- 2-3 servings daily of meat, poultry, fish, eggs, legumes and soy.
- Use sparingly: milk, cheese, fats, oils and sweets.

HOW MUCH IS A SERVING?

The simplest strategy to follow is: "One tablespoon of each type of food for every year of the child's age." (National Network for Child Care, NNCC). Remember, offer a variety of healthy foods and your children will eat what they need. NEVER force your kids to finish what's on their plates if they don't want to.

▼ NUTRITION AFFECTS LEARNING

New research suggests that nutritionally deprived children tend to be less physically active, less curious, less attentive, less independent and more anxious. When children miss meals, they tend to be irritable, disinterested in learning, nervous and unable to concentrate.

THE CHILD WHO EATS POORLY LOSES INTEREST QUICKLY, LACKS ENERGY, IS SICK MORE OFTEN AND IRRITABLE.

ATHLETIC KIDS

Young athletes have high energy needs. A good nutrition program will allow these athletes to improve their performance.

Parents, never let your children skip breakfast! Remember, the energy for an afternoon practice session begins in the morning!

> "Laziness is nothing more than a habit of resting before you get tired."
> — Jules Renard (1864-1910)

ACTIVE INDIVIDUALS

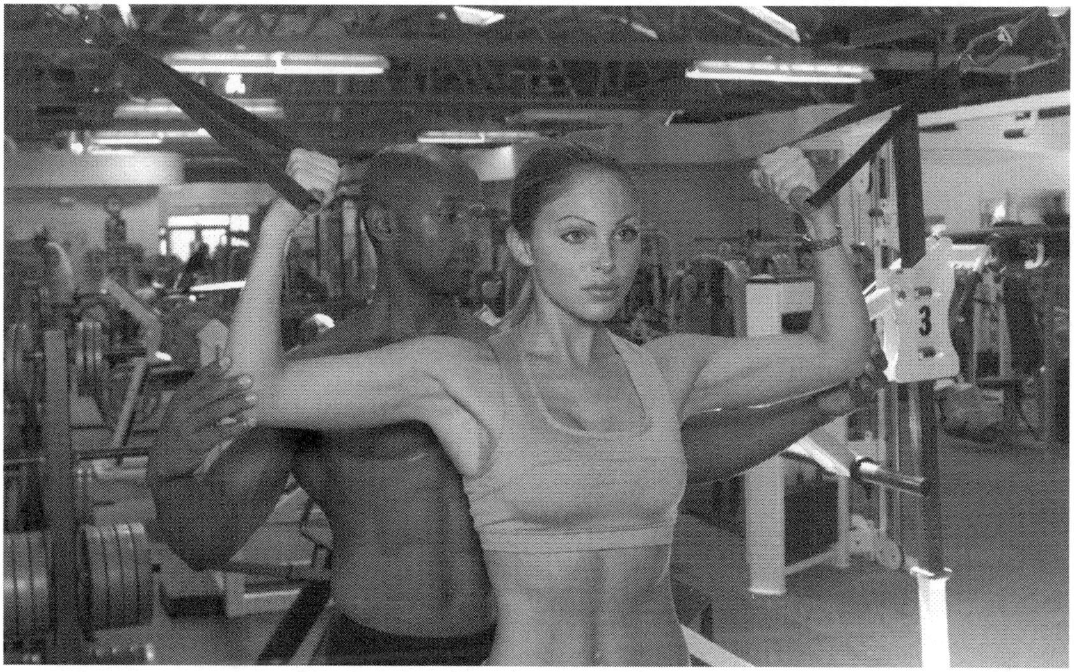

▼ WHY ACTIVE INDIVIDUALS NEED WHOLE FOOD SUPPLEMENTATION

REMOVAL OF TOXINS

We discussed earlier that the body needs the proper balance of amino acids to build and repair muscle and other tissue. Many of these amino acids require certain vitamins and minerals in order to do their jobs. The amino acid Methionine assists in the removal of toxins from the liver and helps to regenerate liver and kidney tissue. It cannot function without vitamin B6 and magnesium. L-carnitine enables your muscle cells to use oxygen more efficiently. It is manufactured through the combination of the amino acid lysine with vitamin C. In a perfect world, you should get your vitamins and minerals from fruits and vegetables. But among the imperfections in our world are the pesticides and preservatives in our food—not to mention the difficulty that most people have eating all the fruits and vegetables they require anyhow, so it's a good idea to supplement your diet with fruit and vegetable capsules. I'm not talking about your everyday vitamin supplements, but we'll discuss this later in this section.

OXIDATIVE STRESS

One of the paradoxes of life is that we need oxygen to sustain life, however, it is also the primary culprit in many diseases (aging, arthritis, cancer, Lou Gehrig's disease, etc.) and degenerative conditions (Marx, 1985).

In normal everyday metabolism, water reacts with oxygen producing a very toxic molecule in our bodies called hydrogen peroxide…a known free radical.

What are free radicals?

Free radicals are vandals and thieves…unstable molecules that roam around in your body burning the cells they come in contact with, trying to steal an electron from those perfectly healthy cells. The science of free radical pathology tells us that the stress on your cells (heart, kidney, lungs, joints, etc.) caused by free radical activity is what leads to aging and many known diseases.

As I mentioned before, normal metabolism—the process by which your body converts the food you eat into usable energy (ATP) for your cells—produces large numbers of free radicals—hydrogen peroxide. We're not talking about a handful of these culprits —each cell in your body produces "one to three billion free radicals per day." [Richard DuBois, MD, Oxidative Stress in the Pathogenesis of Disease and aging; Opportunity for Intervention] In addition, the higher the activity level of an athlete, the more free radicals that are produced.

What does this mean?

It means that active people and high level athletes produce more free radicals than non-active people, consequently causing more stress and damage to the body's tissues and organs. Therefore, the more active you are, the more nutrients your body needs. Don't use this as an excuse to vegetate; there is an easy antidote.

Incidentally, the same formula applies to any kind of stress. The more stressed you are, the more free radicals your body produces.

▼ HOW CAN YOU PREVENT FREE RADICAL DAMAGE TO YOUR CELLS?

Research shows that 6-10 servings of "fresh raw fruits and vegetables" EVERYDAY provide the body with the needed "antioxidants" to "neutralize" free radicals and protect your cells from such oxidative damage.

"Knowing others is wisdom;

Knowing yourself is enlightenment."

—LAO-TZU

What are antioxidants?
Antioxidants are a group of organic substances (vitamin C, E and A, selenium and a group of Carotenoids) found in fruits and vegetables that combine with free radical molecules, converting them back into stable oxygen molecules, thereby preventing cell damage.

THE PROBLEM

Do you eat 6-10 servings of raw fruits and vegetables EVERYDAY? I don't think so! Nobody does. That is where smart supplementation with "whole food" supplements will play a vital role in your athletic performance, your ability to recover from injuries and your overall health and well-being. I'm not suggesting here that you run out and buy antioxidant supplements. They don't work! Research shows that the **best results** come from the **synergistic effect of all the nutrients working together** as they do in nature.

What I recommend:
Find a "whole food concentrate" in capsule form. Clever manufacturers have dehydrated fruits and vegetables, eliminated the sugar and the sodium, and kept all the good stuff that you need—like enzymes, fiber, vitamins, minerals and all the other micro-nutrients both known and "unknown." I say "unknown," because there are a lot of nutrients in fruits and vegetables that we currently don't know anything about since they haven't been associated with any disease.

What should you look for in "whole food supplements?"

The juicing and dehydration process must be done at very *controlled temperatures* so that the nutrients are neither heated nor frozen which would destroy them. Only when these conditions are met will the nutrients from these supplements be "bio-available" to the body—this means that they are readily absorbed into your bloodstream. Clinical research has shown us that this type of whole food supplement is far superior to fragmented vitamin pills that contain random amounts of nutrients. I think nature knows best!

Who are these companies?

NSA markets JuicePlus+®, a product supported by independent clinical research. There is also JuicePower™ by New Vision. To learn more, please visit the nutrition page on my website at www.personalfitness.com.

If you have a specific condition, talk to your doctor, registered dietitian or healthcare practitioner. Otherwise, the only other supplement I recommend is a good protein powder or meal replacement shake. I have my clients use the Jay Robb, Egg White Protein Powder and the JuicePlus+® Complete meal replacement with soy protein. (Ladies, remember that soy contains specific Isoflavones that are beneficial to your specific health needs.) Both of these products are 100% natural with no artificial additives, preservatives or fillers. For those with compromised immune functions, ImmunoProRx™ and GlutImmune™ may also be beneficial. Both are marketed by a company called Biomolecular Sciences.

"Food is an important part of a balanced diet."

— Fran Lebowitz

I've done the research, and I hate to tell you, but everybody dies
- lovers, joggers, vegetarians, and non-smokers.
I'm telling you this so that some of you who jog at five am and eat vegetables
will occassionally sleep late and have an ice cream cone.

— Bernie S. Siegel, M.D.

AMERICA'S SILENT KILLERS

Surprise, surprise

I've got a bubble butt, a wondergut and thunder thighs

Don't know how I got this way

Could it be the burgers and fries?

▼ HYDROGENATED OILS AND TRANS-FATTY ACIDS

Hydrogenated oils and trans-fatty acids are silent killers. Research studies show conclusively that they cause diseases such as non-insulin dependent type II diabetes. Numerous research studies have shown how harmful these oils are to the human body. Hydrogenation of oils acts as a preservative. This leads to increased shelf life and less spoilage of products. But at what cost to the human body?

During the process of hydrogenation, hydrogen atoms are literally moved to the opposite side of the double bond, thereby changing the molecular structure of the fatty acid in the oil. (Fats break down in the body into fatty acids, remember?) This newly formed molecular configuration of the fatty acid, which the genetics of the body does not recognize, has been named "trans," meaning "on the other side of." Trans-fatty acids alter the normal transport of important nutrients across cell membranes. They also weaken the protective structure and function of the cell.

This changed essential fatty acid, which has now become a trans-fatty acid, has the same molecular structure of stearic acid, which is used to make candles hard. If stearic acid can make candles hard, don't you think that in the human body it can cause hardening of the arteries? Hundreds of research studies show conclusively that this is in fact the case. One such14-year study — involving 85,000 nurses — was published by Dr. Walter Willett, Chairman of Nutrition at Harvard Medical. His study clearly shows that people consuming the most trans-fatty acids have the highest rate of heart disease. Period!

Where do you find hydrogenated oils? French fries, fried chicken, vegetable oils, bacon, donuts, chips, canned soups, crackers and cookies — in almost ALL commercially processed foods and at all fast food restaurants.

Research Studies Show these Effects of Trans-Fatty Acids on the Body

(1) Lowers the "good" HDL cholesterol;

(2) Raises the "bad" LDL cholesterol;

(3) Lowers the amount of cream (volume) in milk from lactating women, thus lowering the overall quality available to the infant;

(4) Correlates to low birth weight in human infants;

(5) Affects immune response by lowering efficiency of B cell response and increasing proliferation of T cells;

(6) Decreases levels of testosterone in male animals, increases level of abnormal sperm, and interferes with gestation in females;

(7) Increases breast cancer in women;

(8) Increases heart disease in men and women;

(9) Increases non-insulin dependent type diabetes disease.

▼ ASPARTAME

There is currently a great debate taking place over the safety of aspartame, the sweetener used in most "sugarless" drinks and foods. Some research data claim that aspartame causes brain tumors and uterine polyps in experimental animals. However, the FDA and other scientific bodies disagree.

In my opinion, it doesn't matter who is right. The very fact that there is conflicting research is enough for me. I'm not willing to be a monkey in a scientist's lab. Are you?

Have you heard the latest about Hormone Replacement Therapy? Turns out that after decades of saying it is safe, long term research studies have recently concluded that it increases women's risks for breast cancer, heart disease, strokes and blood clots in the lungs. How could science have been so wrong? Well, to answer this one, you would have to look at who was funding most of the research — drug and pharmaceutical companies.

I would highly recommend that instead of using artificial sweeteners and plastic man-made fats (margarine), use a little natural organic sugar, honey, stevia and real butter. Used in moderation, these will be healthier for you in the long run because the body does not recognize the artificial replacements.

Why would you replace something that nature gave us, like natural sugar cane, for something produced in a laboratory? It doesn't make sense to me — I think nature knows best!

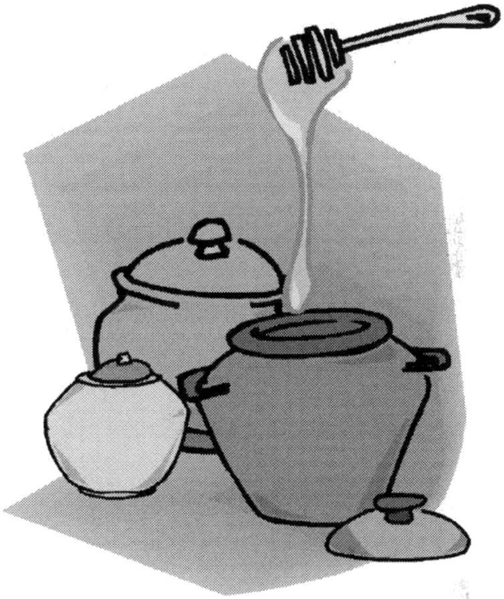

Every 3 minutes a woman is diagnosed with breast cancer, and every twelve minutes a woman dies of it.
Get checked regularly and practice preventive nutrition.

5 KEYS TO SUPERCHARGING YOUR METABOLISM

DEFINITIONS:

Metabolism — the process by which your body converts food into usable cellular energy.

Metabolic Rate — the speed at which metabolism occurs.

(1) LIFT WEIGHTS

Muscles are metabolically active; fat isn't.

(2) DO INTERVAL AEROBIC EXERCISE

Do 30-60 minutes DAILY! Not once or twice per week, DAILY!

Why interval? Your body will respond better when challenged.

(3) ALWAYS EAT BREAKFAST

Skipping breakfast sends your body into starvation mode which slows down your metabolic rate.

(4) NEVER EAT FEWER CALORIES THAN YOUR BMR

Your Basal Metabolic Rate (BMR) is the amount of calories your body needs just to keep you alive (Add a zero to your best weight).

(5) BECOME SUPER ACTIVE

I don't mean you should exercise 24 hours per day. Just make activity the norm in your life. Park farther than usual and walk. Take the stairs. Take a 10 minute walking break instead of that coffee break. Do some push-ups or crunches before going to bed.

> "Eighty percent of success is showing up."
> — Woody Allen

DEL'S BODY TRANSFORMATION PROGRAM

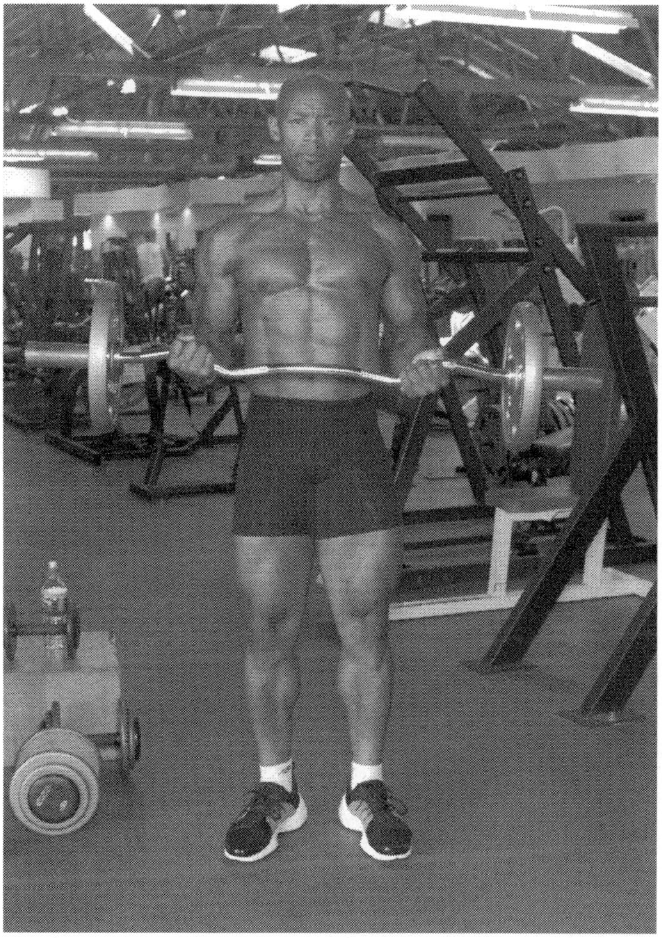

"It takes courage to grow up and turn out to be who you really are."
— E.E. CUMMINGS

Over the past ten years, the vast majority of clients I have worked with have all shared one common goal: **Body Transformation.**

Here's the most important thing to understand:

HEALTH, FITNESS AND

BODY TRANSFORMATION

ARE THREE COMPLETELY

DIFFERENT THINGS.

Why, you may ask? Two reasons:
1. You can be healthy and not fit;
2. You can be fit and fat.

If you're trying to change your body, start by working on your health. This means start making healthier food and lifestyle choices. Notice the word "lifestyle." Health is a lifestyle!

Next, follow a fitness and nutrition program designed to help you change your level of fitness. Before you can work on transforming your body, you must first condition your body to tolerate more intense training. If you've never exercised before or are coming off a long hiatus, this process may take one to two months. Once you've developed a basic level of conditioning, you're ready to take it to the next level: Body Transformation.

Take note of the progression of your program. First, we work on your health. Next your level of fitness, then body transformation. Success is a process, not an event!

Keep in mind that it is impossible to transform your body and not transform your life! Body transformation is a process of transforming your life to create balance! You can make changes to your eating and exercise habits. However, change is temporary! Transformation is forever! Once you've transformed your body and your life, there is no way you can go back to being the way you were. You have expanded your vision of who you think you are, what you're capable of, and how you see yourself. Once you have become conscious of the possibilities for your life, it is almost impossible to go back to sleep! *The pain of slipping back into the darkness becomes far greater than the effort it takes to stay awake!*

"Change is temporary. Transformation is forever!"

> "I love exercise, I could watch it all day long."
> — Bill Russell

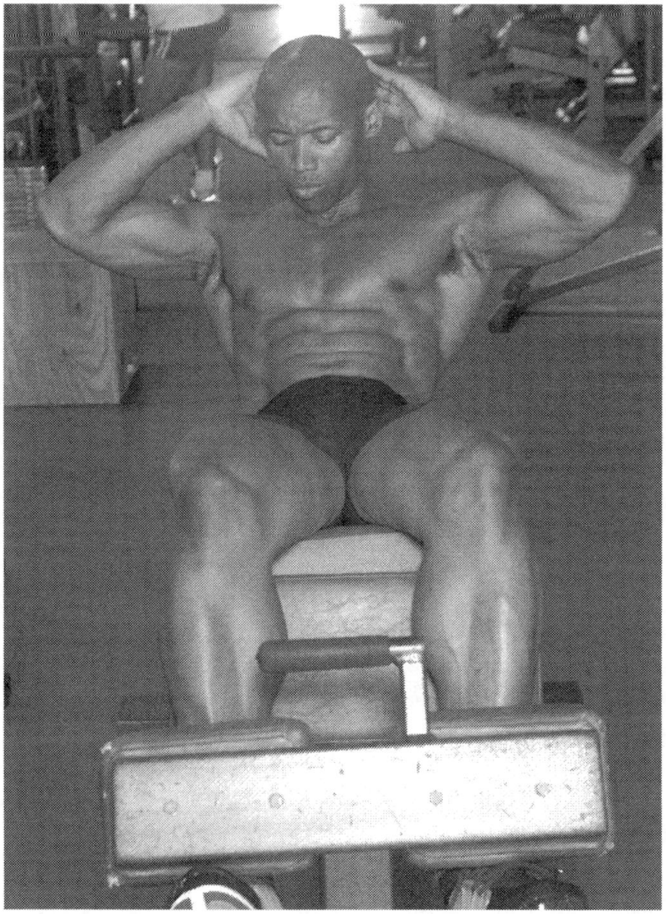

ENTERING THE WINNERS CIRCLE: DESIRE, DISCIPLINE, DETERMINATION!

"A great flame follows a little spark"
— Dante, The Divine Comedy

I have worked with many clients who have transformed their bodies and their lives. I have also worked with others who are still struggling. Success requires: desire, discipline and determination. You must have a very strong desire for what you want. Almost to the point of obsession. Your desire should be so strong that it keeps you up at night, gets you up early in the morning and keeps your eyes burning with future possibilities throughout the day! It is the BIG WHY you will need to keep yourself going when you're tired and exhausted and you're not sure you want to take another step. It is the fuel for your "dream-wagon." Without it, all is lost!

DESIRE is the fuel for your "dream-wagon."

Desire alone, however, will never get you anywhere! Success requires ACTION! Whenever you take one step forward, what you desire is brought two steps toward you. This is important; remember this! You must develop the discipline to stay on course, to follow your plan! If you fall, get up, dust yourself off and keep on going. The truth is you will fall; we all do. Success isn't about who made it without falling. Success is granted to those who fall time and time again but who get up again and again and again! This requires great discipline.

DISCIPLINE is knowing what you have to do to get a desired outcome and being totally committed to doing it...whether you feel like it or not!

"Your own resolution to success is more important than any other one thing."
—Abraham Lincoln

The final piece of the master plan is determination. Determination is the "will" to bend the forces of the universe to your calling. When you are determined, the very thing you seek becomes a dance between life and death. Death, of course, is not an option; therefore, the only possibility is to LIVE! To succeed!

DETERMINATION is an "iron will" whose mantra is: "Success is Imminent! Failure is not an option!"

Remember, change is temporary. Transformation is forever! To transform your body and your life, you must have desire, discipline and determination! When you possess these three critical elements, success is imminent! Welcome to the Winners Circle!

"Whatever you can do, or dream you can, begin it. Boldness has genius, power, and magic in it. Begin it now!
— Goethe

DESTINY

Destiny is not a road for the weak-hearted
First it takes Desire just to get started
Then it takes Discipline and a sense of self control
Finally Determination to get you to your goal

But if you have the Desire you'll find your way somehow
The sound you hear is Destiny calling, the time to start is Now!

▼ YOUR ROADMAP

You can have all the desire, discipline and determination in the world, but without a good plan, your success may be unduly delayed. So, here's the plan in its simplicity:

IDENTIFY SPECIFICALLY HOW YOU WANT TO SEE YOUR BODY CHANGE. If you need to lose or gain weight, how much and why? What dress size or waist size will you be? What do you look like when you have successfully transformed your body. Describe yourself in vivid details. You must be able to see it—and even feel it—before you can achieve it!

HOW WILL THIS CHANGE YOUR LIFE?
What will you have that you don't already have?

WHY IS THIS IMPORTANT TO YOU?
WHY, WHY, WHY? This is your BIG WHY that will help you get up and get back on track when you fall down. Remember, you will stumble, and you will fall; we all do. However, sometimes in order to get up we have to remind ourselves WHY we must!

WHAT CHALLENGES WILL YOU FACE?
How will you use them as learning experiences? If there weren't any challenges, you would already have what you desire.

NEXT, YOU NEED A FITNESS AND NUTRITION PROGRAM.

➤ THE FITNESS PLAN

3 Days of weight training
3-5 Days cardiovascular (brisk walking, jogging, biking, stairmaster, aerobics, etc.)

I recommend that you find a fitness professional in your area who can design a weight training program for you, especially if you're new at it.

➤ YOUR NUTRITION PLAN

A. Your nutrition plan should consist of **4-6 regular meals each day**, every 3-4 hours. Notice I did say "meals" not "snacks." Get in the habit of eating balanced meals, with a serving of protein the size of your palm and a serving of carbohydrates the size of your fist; include a serving of vegetables with at least two of your meals.

B. **Keep a daily food and exercise journal**. You want to be able to identify exactly what you're doing a month down the road. You don't want to be playing guessing games. If your progress slows, your journal will quickly identify areas in which you may be slacking off. You want to be honest with yourself.

C. **Drink 10-12 glasses of water everyday. Every day!**

D. **Maintain your plan for six days out of the week and have one free day**. On your free day, eat WHATEVER YOU WANT. Treat yourself! Remember, *if you do something once a week, it's a treat; if you do it 2-3 times a week, it's a habit.* Habits either take you closer to your goals, or they keep you right where you are.

E. **Ask yourself regularly, "Is what I'm eating taking me closer to my goal?"** If it does, continue eating it. If it doesn't, make a better choice.

EVALUATE YOUR PROGRESS MONTHLY AND REWARD YOURSELF FOR YOUR ACCOMPLISHMENTS.

If it seems like nothing is happening, review your food and exercise log. Ask yourself, "on a scale of 1-10, how committed am I to my plan?"

You are born small and weak.
You die small and weak.
How you look in between is up to you.
—Designer Protein (advertisement)

DEL'S LIFE TRANSFORMATION TIPS

HERE ARE A FEW THINGS TO CONSIDER:

- There are more diets available for people to follow today, yet Americans are fatter than ever. And the rest of the world is following closely behind because the American fast food empire is no longer just an American tragedy, it is now a global disaster!

- With that said, you should also know that every fad diet on the market today will help you to successfully "lose weight." Really! They're not lying! What they're not telling you is that most of that weight will be water and lean muscle tissue. The two most important things your body is made of. And the two things you don't want to lose.

- Remember, transformation is a process! And you cannot transform your body without also transforming your life! So, if the plan that I've outlined for you above is too lofty a goal, then why not set yourself up to succeed by focusing on one new change at a time. Here's what it looks like:

CHANGE #1 — Exercise for 10 minutes a day for one week.

That's 70 minutes of exercise you've done that you weren't doing before. At the end of a month that's 300 minutes. At the end of one year that's 3650 minutes of exercise you're now doing — that's over 60 hours! If you don't know what to do, get a copy of my book, Del's 10 minute Totally Body Workout. Will it make a difference? You bet your unclogged arteries it will! Keep in mind that:

> "Big transformation comes from doing small things consistently over time! It's the little things that will eventually make the BIG difference!"

CHANGE #2—Pick one meal, any meal, and focus on making it the most healthy and nutritious meal of your day — according to my nutrition guidelines in the latter part of the book. Make it the same meal everyday for one week. My recommendation is to choose the meal that is the most challenging for you. If you usually skip breakfast, choose breakfast. Do you usually run to a fast food restaurant for lunch? If so, choose lunch. If all your meals are equally as challenging, just choose one.

CHANGE #3— Choose another meal and focus on it everyday for one week. It is important to note that at the end of each week you're not discontinuing what you've been focusing on, you're just adding a new habit.

CHANGE #4— Drop everything you're doing and take a 10 minute walk every day. Here are some suggestions…

- Walk to and from lunch.
- If you have meetings everyday with one or two people, why not have a walking meeting, instead of the stale old sitting in the office.
- Instead of the coffee break, go for a walk around the neighborhood.
- If you work from home, force yourself to go walk around the block as you return those phone calls or check your voicemail.

Cumulatively, at the end of your first month, here's what you're doing:

- You're exercising everyday.
- You're eating at least two healthy nutritious meals everyday.
- You're taking stress breaks during your day, everyday.

At the end of your first month, continue adding small weekly changes and at the end of one year, your life will have been given an upgrade! Remember what I said earlier about big transformation comes about by making small changes consistently over time?

CONGRATULATIONS!!
YOUR LIFE HAS BEEN TRANSFORMED!!

Before we go on to the recipe part of the book, let's see if you've been paying attention. To find out, here's DR. DEL's QUIZ:

DR. DEL'S QUIZ

- Every organ and tissue in your body is made of microscopic cells. Where does your body get the raw material to build those cells?
  a) Trader Joes; b) DNA; c) food

- What is the major element in muscle?

- What does the Aquarian carry?

- What does the Sahara not have enough of, and Seattle have too much of?
  If your answer to all three is coffee, then go back and reread pages ?-?.

- To build lean muscle mass drink every day at least:
  a) 10 Dr.Diet Pepper's; b) 6 Tuna smoothies; c) 1 gallon of water

- Fill in the blank: "If you don't eat the right foods today, you will end up wearing _________________ tomorrow!"
  a) John Goodman's old clothes, b) a permanent frown, c) the wrong ones

- Which of the following statements is true?
  a) no news is always good news; b) all Italians are basically the same;
  c) all carbohydrates are not basically the same

- Simple sugars are:
  a) chocolate bars without nuts; b) carbohydrates found in candies, fruit, fruit juices, syrups, etc; c) white and granulated and they come in little packages at Dennys

- From a sugar standpoint, a glass of orange juice is no different than:
  a) a can of regular cola; b) a can of motor oil; c) a week in Detroit

- Fill in the blank: The Anaerobic Energy System is the primary source of muscle energy for exercise that lasts:
  a) less than 10 seconds; b) up to 3 minutes; c) all night long

- Fat serves a vital purpose in your body.
  a) it helps you avoid being in an intimate relationship; b) it makes you humble;
  c) it protects your organs, provides vitamins and is necessary for hormonal production.

- The amount of fat your body burns during exercise depends upon your level of cardiovascular fitness and:
  a) the tightness of your workout clothes; b) the temperature of the room; c) your percentage of lean muscle mass

- Which burns the most fat calories?
  a) walking on a treadmill at low intensities; b) walking on a treadmill at higher intensities; c) walking on a treadmill without plugging it in

- The saying **M**y **G**randmother **L**ikes **N**uts and **S**eeds is:
  a) my way of telling you that my grandfather was a nut; b) my grandmother was a squirrel; c) a simple food combining formula

- If you exercise while your body is in starvation mode:
  a) you will break down your muscle tissue; b) you'll definitely lose a lot of weight; c) you could receive the Mahatmas Gandhi Award

- Which two of the following does not belong in the list?
  The amount of calories you need daily depends on the following factors:
  Your age, weight, height, percent body fat, your ability to do simple addition, whether you eat standing up or sitting down, fitness goals.

- One of the following statements is true:
  a) you've got to be fat to lose fat; b) you've got to hate fat to lose fat; c) you've got to eat fat to lose fat

- To lose fat weight:
  a) reduce daily calories by 15-20%; b) go on the famous Cumquat Diet of the Stars; c) only eat on alternate Thursdays

- 1 in 4 children in the US today:
  a) is ambidextrous; b) will end up working at Starbucks; c) is seriously overweight

- Health, fitness and body transformation are basically the same.
  True or false?

- Which statement is not true:
  a) you can be healthy and not fit; b) you can be fit and fat; c) you can be fat and skinny

- How many servings of fresh raw fruits and vegetables should you consume daily?
a) one is enough if you eat the rinds, skins, stems and pits; b) none, as fruits and vegetables don't have enough preservatives; c) 6-10

- Never skip:
a) rope; b) dessert ; c) breakfast

- Free radicals are:
a) revolutionaries out on parole; b) liberal thinkers who don't wear underwear or seat belts ;c) unstable molecules that roam around in your body

- Since active people and high level athletes produce more free radicals than non-active people:
a) they must make sure that they have enough antioxidants to neutralize the free radicals; b) they must register with the US Free Radical Governing Board; c) they must not only succeed at their activity, but then they must get out of town

- A Cambridge University study found that people who participate in vigorous activities are less likely to suffer from:
a) agoraphobia; b) hip fractures; c) amnesia

- While you are sleeping:
a) your body builds and repairs muscle tissue; b) your body astral projects to Jamaica, returning just before the alarm goes off; c) somebody is filling out your daily planner

- Which of the following is not one of my Five Keys to Supercharge your Metabolism?
a) lift weights; b) do interval aerobic exercise; c) always eat breakfast; d) talk as fast as you can; e) become super active

- *Which doesn't belong in this list?* Success requires:
a) desire; b) discipline; c) determination; d) dinero

- In my fitness plan, you have a free day every week. On this free day:
a) don't eat anything; b) only eat food beginning with the letter "f"; c) eat whatever you want

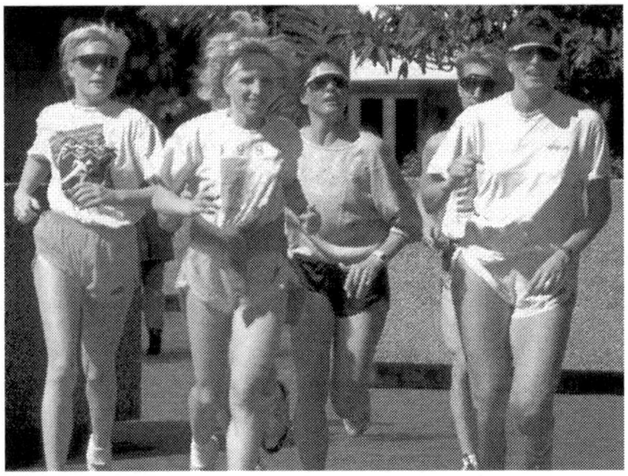

Learn to work harder on yourself
than you do on your job.

— Jim Rohn

FREQUENTLY ASKED QUESTIONS

FREQUENTLY ASKED QUESTIONS ABOUT EXERCISE AND NUTRITION:

When does the body start to burn fat?
Your body is always burning fat. You burn fat while you're sitting in front of the television set and during exercise. Of course you burn more fat during exercise because the body's energy demands increase. With the exception of very high intensity exercise, your body is always burning fat. And no, it is not true that it takes 30-40 minutes to start burning fat.

If I only workout for ten minutes, is it doing me any good and am I burning any fat?
Recent scientific studies confirm that short bouts of exercise are just as effective for improving your fitness level as longer sessions. So, if you only have 10 minutes to spare, why not follow along with one of the 10 minute workouts in my book, *Del's 10 minute Total Body Workout.* Remember, 10 minutes per day every day adds up to almost 5 hours each month. Is that better than doing nothing at all? You bet it is. Will it help you to burn more fat? Why don't you get off the couch and find out?

How do I get rid of the cellulite on my thighs?
Let's talk about cellulite. What exactly is cellulite? Cellulite is not really a function of how much excess weight or fat you have on your body. In fact, it is nothing more than an irregular pattern of connective tissue beneath the skin. And when your fatty tissue, which forms in little honeycomb compartments, pushes against the skin, it causes dimpling, which women call cellulite. This is a genetic condition and skin creams will only make your skin swell so that the appearance of the cellulite changes, but the effects are only temporary. Your best bet is to follow a good exercise and nutrition program to lose excess body fat.

Which exercises burn the most fat?
When people ask me this question, I realize that they really don't have an understanding of how the fat burning process works. If you're trying to lose weight, your primary objective is to burn more calories than you consume. Therefore, it really doesn't matter which exercises you do to a certain extent...your goal is to burn as many calories as possible and every exercise burns calories. However, do keep in mind that weight training builds muscles and the more muscles you have on your body the more fat you will burn. So, here's the bottom-line, do some weight training, some cardiovascular activity, have a great nutrition program and become super-ac-

tive.

How much muscle do I lose when I lose weight?

Research tells us that up to 25% of weight loss can be from lean muscle tissue. Chances are if you lose a lot of weight over a short period of time, most of that weight will be water and lean muscle, not fat. To minimize muscle loss and maximize fat loss, lose weight slowly (1-2 lbs./ week), get on a weight training program to build lean muscle, and supplement your diet with a fruit and vegetable concentrate (like JuicePlus+®), glutamine and EFA's.

Can eating too much fructose actually slow the fat burning process?

Fructose is the simple sugar found in fruit. Studies confirm that the presence of sugar in the bloodstream during exercise will actually slow the fat-burning process dramatically. For this reason, I always recommend working out on an empty stomach. Keep in mind that we're talking about aerobic activity, since this is the primary way your body can metabolize fatty acids.

Why is it a bad idea to cut fats from my diet?

The problem with low fat diets is that every cell, tissue, gland and organ in your body needs fat in order to function. There are two important fatty acids your body cannot make; therefore, these must be supplied via your diet—these are what we call *essential fatty acids* (EFA's)—omega-3 and omega-6 fatty acids. EFA's are responsible for a host of critical functions in the body such as sperm formation, heart function, how well your cells absorb nutrients, and visual functions. They also increase testosterone production, optimize thyroid function and are also anti-inflammatory. Most people on a low-fat diet do not get an adequate supply of EFA's, therefore will actually find it more difficult to lose weight and gain muscle.

Will I burn more fat if I exercise on an empty stomach?

To optimize your fat burning, the best time to exercise is first thing in the morning on an empty stomach. At this time your body is starved for carbohydrates and is forced to use fat for energy. The evening is also a good time, three hours after your afternoon meal or snack. Why are these the best times? A research team from the University of Texas reported that subjects burned almost twice as much fat when they exercised on an empty stomach than those who had 60 grams of carbohydrates an hour prior to exercise. This does not apply to weight training. If you're training to build muscle and strength, you may actually benefit from a carbohydrate drink before or during your workout.

Can eating more fats increase my IQ?

Researchers say that eating more essential fatty acids not only speeds learning but can also increase your IQ by 6-9 points.

Can a low-fat diet lead to developmental and behavioral problems in my children?

The research on women and children says that each time a woman has a child she loses about 3% of her brain weight that must be replaced. Each child she has depletes her further and each also gets less essential fatty acids than the previous one—this is why, on average, older children have the highest IQ in the family. Since the brain is over 60% fat, it is important to have a good source of EFA's in your diet especially during pregnancy.

How can eating more fats help me to lose weight?

Let's qualify what kinds of fats we're talking about. Saturated and hydrogenated fats will kill you. However, essential fatty acids, especially the omega-3 fatty acids found in flaxseed oil, inhibit fat production in the body by limiting the activity of genes that make enzymes required for fat production. Omega-3 fatty acids also improve the function of the genes that make enzymes required for fat burning and increase the body's metabolic rate by increasing thermogenesis—heat production. To get a good balance of both omega-3 and omega-6 fatty acids, add some salmon, trout and flax seed oil to your daily diet.

Is interval training more effective for fat burning than walking at a steady pace?

The answer is yes! Several research studies have demonstrated the superiority of one minute interval training in fat loss. Even if you were to burn the same amount of calories, studies show that higher intensity exercise may further aid weight loss due to an acute increase in energy expenditure up to 24 hours following exercise. Another reason to up the intensity is that it will increase your level of fitness. The fitter you are the more effective your body will be at burning fat.

A University of Illinois study found that frozen produce retains up to twice as many vitamins as unfrozen produce that has spent a few days in the store or refrigerator.

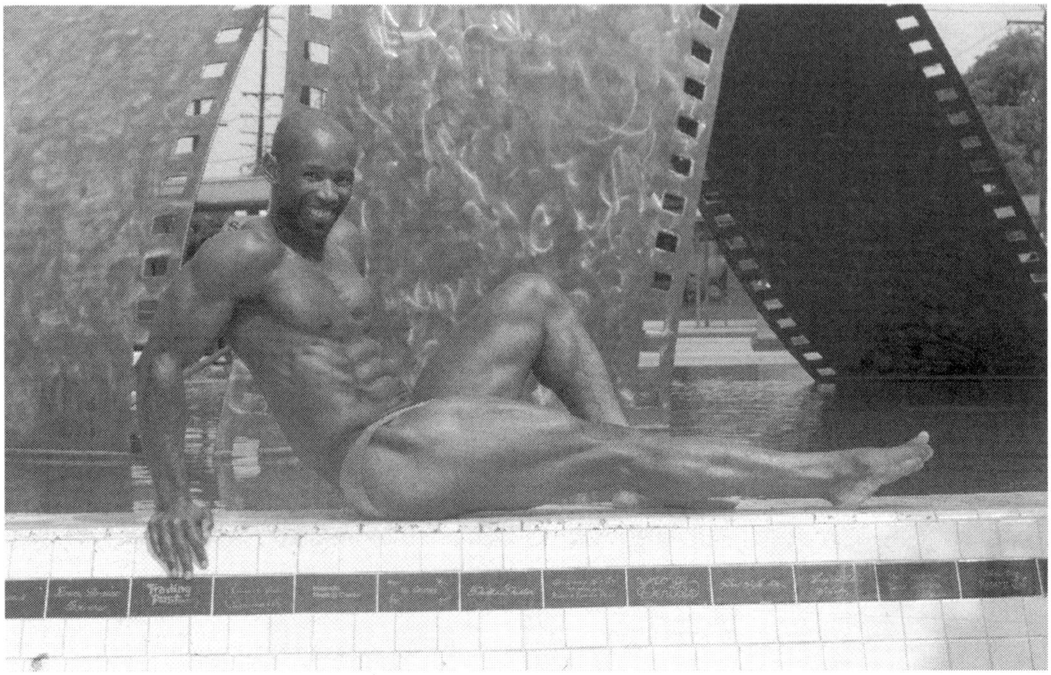

SUCCESS STRATEGY:

Strive for consistency, not perfection.

It's a given that you will stray from your nutrition plan, whatever that plan is. When you do, enjoy it, then recommit to your plan with your next meal.

DEL'S SUGGESTED FOOD LIST

PROTEINS

Chicken breast

Turkey breast

Lean ground chicken, turkey or beef

Egg whites

Salmon or trout

Orange roughy

Water packed white albacore canned tuna

Low-fat cottage cheese

Buffalo

Lamb

VEGETARIAN PROTEINS

Tofu

Tempeh

Seitan

Soy products

Veggie burgers

CARBOHYDRATES

Baked yam

Fruits

Oatmeal

Legumes

Steamed brown or wild rice

Vegetables

Whole wheat bread

Corn

Fat-free plain yogurt

FATS

Avocado

Flax seed oil

Extra-virgin olive oil

Canola oil

Natural peanut butter

Fats to AVOID:

Butter or margarine

Fried foods

Whole milk and whole milk products

Mayonnaise

A Cambridge University study found that people who participate in vigorous activities are less likely to suffer from hip fractures.

If you're like most of my clients, you're trying to change your body or at the very least maintain the fitness level that you've worked very hard to attain. It is important to combine protein and carbohydrates at each meal to feed your growing muscles and to give your body enough energy for your activities. Eat a small meal every three to four hours (4-6 small meals daily), with a portion of protein that fits in the palm of your hand and carbohydrates the size of your fist. Include a serving of vegetables with at least two of your daily meals.

You will find that each recipe in this book is a complete balanced meal.

Don't forget to drink at least 12 glasses of water EVERY DAY!

Remember, muscle tissue is primarily water, not protein!

▼ YOUR SEVEN DAY SHOPPING LIST

Old fashion oatmeal
Protein powder
Chicken breasts
Cottage cheese
Plain non-fat yogurt
Salmon
Eggs
Cans of tuna
Ground turkey breasts
Ground chicken breasts
Steak
Black beans
Sea bass
Snapper
White beans
Broccoli
Avocado
Ginger
Lentils
Rice
Pasta
Tomatoes
Basil
Fresh fruit and vegetables
Mixed baby salad greens (ReadyPac)
Baby spinach (ReadyPac)

YOUR SEVEN DAY SAMPLE MEAL PLAN

DAY 1

Meal One: Oatmeal with cinnamon and nutmeg; fruit & vegetable capsules (i.e. JuicePlus+®)

Meal Two: Protein smoothie

Meal Three: Chicken w/ broccoli

Meal Four: Cottage cheese & yogurt

Meal Five: Pan-fried salmon; fruit and vegetable capsules

Note 1: Don't forget your 10-12 glasses of water daily.

Note 2: Take your fruit and vegetable capsules prior to your meals. The JuicePlus+® brand contains active enzymes that aid in the digestive process.

DAY 2

Meal One: Breakfast burrito, 1 piece fruit; fruit and vegetable capsules

Meal Two: Protein smoothie

Meal Three: Chicken, avocado & rice salad

Meal Four: Black beans & tuna

Meal Five: Honey mustard snapper, fruit and vegetable capsules

Day 3

Meal One: Banana-oatmeal-egg white pancakes; fruit and vegetable capsules

Meal Two: Protein smoothie

Meal Three: Ground chicken with tomato and basil

Meal Four: Sweet tuna and pasta salad

Meal Five: Mustard baked salmon with lentils, fruit & vegetable capsules

Day 4

Meal One: Scrambled tofu with tomatoes; fruit & vegetable capsules

Meal Two: Protein smoothie

Meal Three: Ginger sesame chicken

Meal Four: White bean turkey chili

Meal Five: Asian-style sea bass; fruit & vegetable capsules

Day 5

Meal One: Scrambled Egg Whites with Tomato, Basil & Avocado; fruit and vegetable capsules

Meal Two: Protein Smoothie

Meal Three: Grilled Chicken Breast Salad

Meal Four: Cottage Cheese Spread

Meal Five: Spicy Fish Tacos; fruit & vegetable capsules

Day 6

Meal One: Hot Oatmeal with Cinnamon and Nutmeg; fruit & vegetable capsules

Meal Two: Protein Smoothie

Meal Three: Steak & Broccoli with Spicy Chili Sauce

Meal Four: Tantalizing Turkey Tacos; fruit & vegetable capsules

Day 7

FREE DAY!! FREE DAY!! TREAT YOURSELF, EAT ANYTHING YOU WANT!! GO FOR BROKE!! DON'T HOLD BACK!! BOOGIE WOOGIE!

> **"Bad habits are like a comfortable bed, easy to get into, but hard to get out of."**
>
> — Unknown

▼ WHAT YOU WILL NEED IN YOUR KITCHEN

THE BASICS:

Pots and pans
A set of knives
A cutting board
A set of measuring spoons
A stove (this would be helpful!)
Hand grater
Wooden spoons
Can opener
Blender
Microwave

FRESH HERBS AND SPICES:

Basil (fresh and dried)
Curry powder
Nutmeg
Ground cinnamon
Oregano
Paprika
Parsley
Thyme
Tumeric
Vanilla extract
Fresh garlic
Onions
Lemon/Lime juice
Salt & pepper
Vinegar (Balsamic & rice wine)
Extra virgin olive oil
Ginger
Dijon mustard
Tamari
Sesame seeds
Mustard seeds
Bragg's Liquid Amino's
Reduced sodium soy sauce
Latin mayonnaise
Low sodium chicken & vegetable stock
Non-fat cooking spray

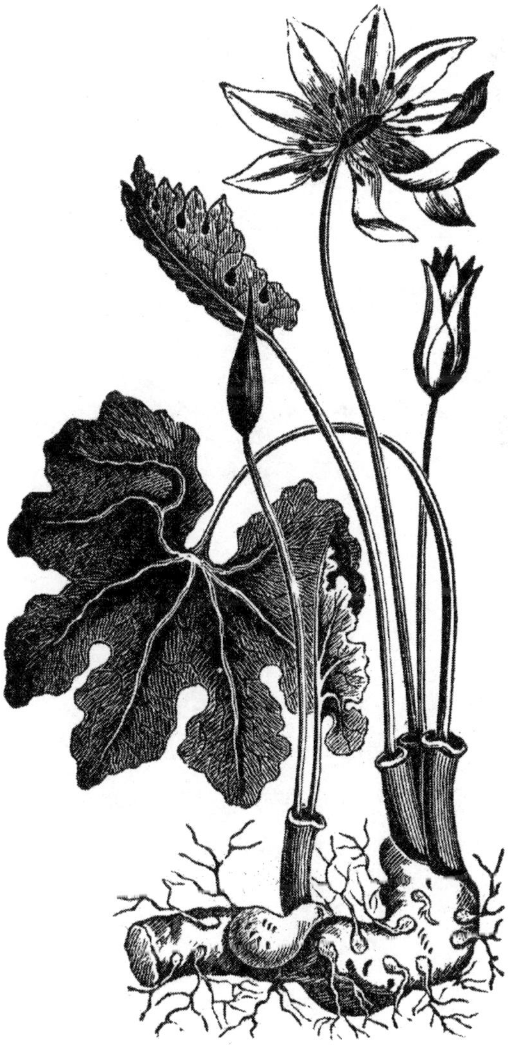

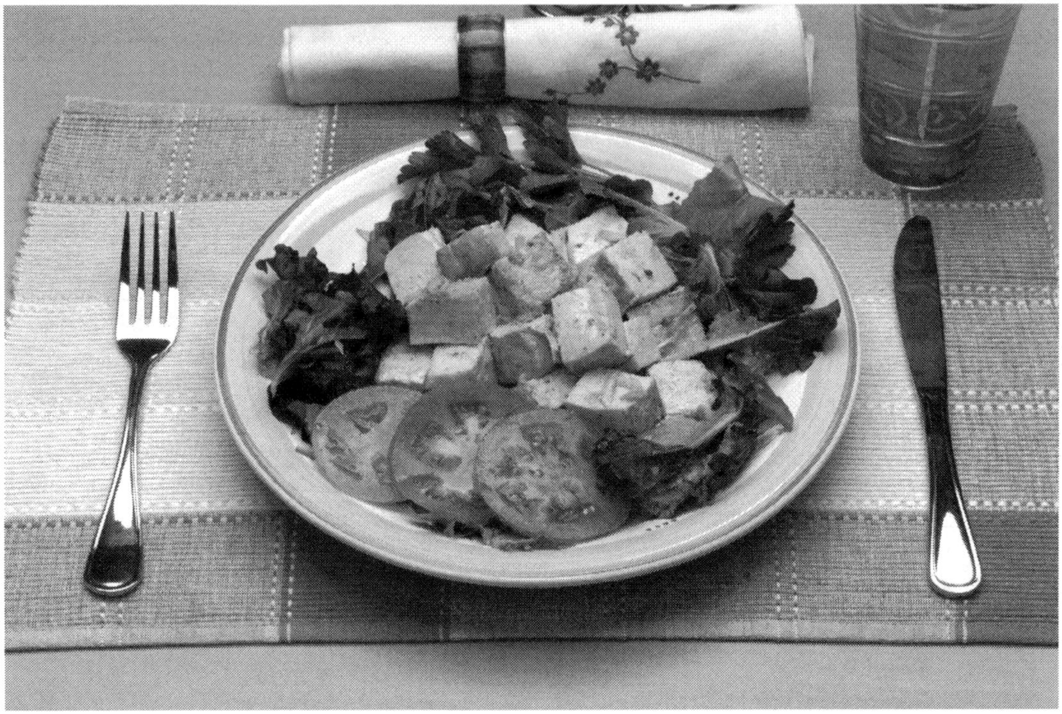

The Antioxidants (Vitamins A, C, E)
help to reduce tissue damage, speed up muscle recovery
and help to build up your immune system.
But forget the pills, make fruits and vegetables
a daily habit, not an occasional occurrence.

TIPS & SUGGESTIONS

TIPS AND SUGGESTIONS FOR SAVING YOURSELF TIME IN THE KITCHEN:

❶ To steam vegetables, put them in a saucepan with 1/2 cup water over medium heat for 5 minutes.

❷ Most vegetables for stir-fry can be found in pre-cut ready to use packages at your local supermarket. I have seen everything from shredded carrots to diced potatoes and everything in between.

❸ Use a variable speed blender or Vitamix machine to chop your vegetables (including onion and garlic) or mince your meat on a low speed. Within a couple minutes, you could chop and mince a couple cups of vegetables and meats, all in your Vitamix machine. If you don't have one, you really need to get one.

❹ Before you do your shopping, choose the recipes you would like to make for the coming week and be sure to buy the necessary ingredients.

❺ VEGETARIANS TAKE NOTE:

You can substitute tempeh, tofu and seitan instead of the chicken, steak, turkey and fish in any of the following recipes. Also, use vegetable stock instead of chicken stock.

TIPS FOR MAKING YOUR OWN MARINADES

Marinades are usually a combination of a juice, vinegar or broth with herbs and spices. Make your own by combining one item from each column below.

1/2 cup	2 tbsp.	1 tsp.	1 tsp.
orange juice	balsamic vinegar	honey	Mrs. Dash & olive oil
lemon juice	red wine vinegar	dijon mustard	Mixed herb blend
Worcestershire sauce	Bragg's Liquid Amino	brown sugar	hot pepper sauce
chicken broth	soy sauce	sweet mustard	curry powder
A-1 or BBQ sauce	tamari sauce	miso	sesame oil, ginger
blended tofu	tahini	sucanat	basil, thyme

quick & easy
10 MINUTE
"FIT" recipes &
nutrition guide

Food that tastes good, and is sooooo nutritious
But it's gotta come quick to be DELicious
Pardon me for seeming a bit repetitious
But it 's gotta be healthy and nutritious
And simple to prepare to be DELicious

So here's what I say to every woman and man
Every girl and boy
Think right, be right, eat right
And whatever you do: ENJOY

- **THE FOLLOWING RECIPES ARE COMPLETE BALANCED MEALS WITH PROTEIN AND CARBOHYDRATES.**

- **I HAVE ALSO MADE NO DISTINCTION BETWEEN BREAKFAST, LUNCH AND DINNER RECIPES.**

- **WHAT I RECOMMEND IS 4-6 SMALL MEALS DAILY EVERY 3-4 HOURS.**

- **EACH RECIPE CAN BE USED TO FULFILL ANY MEAL REQUIREMENT.**

Hot Oatmeal with Cinnamon & Nutmeg

1 cup old fashion oats
1/2 cup vanilla soymilk
1 medium banana, chopped
1 cup water
1 to 2 scoop egg white or soy protein powder
1/2 tsp. cinnamon
1/2 tsp. nutmeg
1 tsp. vanilla extract
2 tsp. honey or sucanat (optional)

❶ Combine oats and water in a pot and let cook for 5 minutes, stirring occasionally.

❷ Stir in soymilk, cinnamon, nutmeg, vanilla extract, honey (optional) and protein powder.*

❸ Serve in a bowl topped with chopped bananas.

*<u>**Note:**</u> Women: 1 scoop protein powder
Men: medium to large build: 2 scoops

<Makes 2 servings>

▼

Yum Yum! I love oatmeal because it reminds me of eating porridge as a boy growing up in Jamaica. Forget the instant stuff and go for the "old fashioned," 100% whole grain type instead. It cooks in only 5 minutes and it has more fiber.

Scrambled Egg Whites with Tomatoes, Basil & Avocado

4 to 8 large free-range egg whites, beaten (discard the yolks)
1 medium tomato, chopped
Mrs. Dash
1 small avocado, chopped
6 fresh basil leafs, chopped
Olive oil or canola oil-based spray
1 bowl chopped fruit

❶ Evenly coat a 10-inch non-stick frying pan with non-fat spray over medium heat.

❷ Sauté tomato and basil for about 1 minute.

❸ Add beaten egg whites and avocado, scramble until firm.

❹ Season to taste.

❺ Serve with a bowl of chopped fruit.

<Makes 1-2 servings>

▼

If you're not used to eating egg whites, it definitely takes getting used to. With the tomato, avocado and basil, you won't miss the yolk. DELicious!!!

Banana Oatmeal Egg-White Pancakes

1/4 cup whole wheat flour
1/2 cup old fashioned oatmeal
1 tsp. baking powder
6 egg whites
3/4 cup soy milk
1/2 tsp. cinnamon
1/2 tsp. nutmeg
1 tsp. vanilla extract
1 medium banana, thinly chopped
Olive oil or canola oil non-fat spray

❶ Combine in a bowl: flour, oats, baking powder, cinnamon, nutmeg.

❷ Combine egg whites, soy milk and vanilla extract in a blender and whip.

❸ Evenly stir blended mixture and chopped bananas in bowl with flour and oats and let sit for 1 minute.

❹ Pour batter onto hot, lightly sprayed griddle or skillet.

❺ Cook until tiny bubbles form on top of pancakes, then turn over (approximately 1-2 minutes on each side).

❻ Serve pancakes hot with fruit preserve.

<Makes 1-2 servings>

▼

Who said you have to give up your favorite foods in order to eat healthy and stay fit? Oatmeal pancakes are the BOMB, BABY!!! They're high in protein and fiber and they taste GREEEAAATTT!!

Strawberries with Almond Cottage Cheese & Yogurt

1 cup fresh strawberries (or other fresh berries)
1 cup low-fat cottage cheese
1/2 cup plain non-fat yogurt
1 tsp. almond extract or vanilla extract
1 tsp. pure cane sugar
1 tsp. thinly sliced almonds

❶ Combine everything except berries and almond in a blender and puree 30 seconds.

❷ Serve on a plate of berries. Garnish cottage cheese mixture with almonds.

<Makes 1-2 servings>

▼

One of my personal training clients actually turned me on to this recipe. I personally don't care much for cottage cheese. I just can't seem to get the phrase "cottage cheese thighs" out of my head. Not to turn you off or anything because it actually is a great source of protein.

Chocolate Peanut Butter Oatmeal

1/2 cup old fashioned oats
1 cup water
1/4 cup vanilla soy milk
1 tsp. natural peanut butter
1 scoop Chocolate JuicePlus+® Complete or other protein powder

❶ Combine oatmeal and water in a pot and cook for 5 minutes over medium heat, stirring occasionally.

❷ Stir in peanut butter until it melts and appears smooth.

❸ Add protein powder and soymilk. Stir and enjoy!

<Makes 1-2 servings>

▼

This is the only way I can get my client Mary to eat oatmeal. Since she loves peanut butter, why not have her oatmeal taste like peanut butter? Brilliant, aren't I? Peanut butter is not the greatest source of fat. However, don't forget that sometimes a little bit of hell makes heaven taste mo-better! If that makes any sense to you!

Breakfast Burrito

2 large whole wheat tortillas
6 egg whites, beaten
1/4 cup shredded low-fat or soy cheese (optional)
1/2 green pepper, chopped
1/2 cup cooked black beans
1/2 onion, chopped
Olive oil or canola oil spray
salt and pepper to taste
2 tbsp. salsa

❶ Evenly spray skillet and sauté onion, pepper and black beans over medium heat.

❷ Add egg whites and cheese, scramble until eggs are cooked.

❸ Warm tortillas according to package directions so they are soft enough to roll.

❹ Place egg mixture along the center of tortillas; top with a tbsp. of salsa and roll up burrito style. Enjoy!

<Makes 1-2 servings>

▼

I came across this recipe from a little health food store called The Farm Store that was right down the street from my home in Culver City, California. Of course they originally used whole eggs but I worked my magic on them and they changed to egg whites. Which reminds me, when you eat out, don't be bashful about asking for what you want…you're paying for it!

Cottage Cheese Spread

1 chopped apple
1/2 tsp. cinnamon
1 cup non-fat cottage cheese
2 slices whole wheat bread, toasted

❶ Combine all ingredients in a bowl (except bread) and microwave for 20-30 seconds.

❷ Spread over whole wheat toast. Enjoy!

<Makes 2 servings>

▼

Someone on my email list shared this recipe with me. If it was you, thanks! Email me and I will give you the credit you deserve next time around. A lot of my clients really like it.

Scrambled Tofu with Tomatoes and Avocado

12 ounces of firm tofu
1/2 medium onion, chopped
1 large fresh tomato, chopped
1/2 large green pepper, chopped
2 cloves fresh garlic, chopped
1 small avocado or 1/2 large, chopped
Mrs. Dash to taste
Olive oil or canola oil non-fat spray

1. Evenly spray a large skillet with non-fat spray.
2. Sauté onion, pepper and garlic for 1 minute.
3. Crush the tofu with a fork. Add tofu, tomatoes and avocado to skillet.
4. Sauté over medium heat for 3 minutes.
5. Add Mrs. Dash to taste and serve.

<Makes 1-2 servings>

▼

I used to HATE tofu until the day I was introduced to really GREAT vegetarian cooking by a wonderful chef at a retreat center in Ojai, California. I didn't know what I was eating and frankly I didn't care. It was just GREAT food...AND for goodness sake, it was tofu! Try this recipe instead of eggs sometimes, or add tofu to your eggs. DELicious!

DELicious SMOOTHIES

Note 1: If you don't already have one, I recommend that you get yourself a Vita-Mix machine. It's one of the best health investments I've ever made!

Note 2: I recommend the JuicePlus+® Complete meal replacement powder, the Jay Robb Egg White protein powder & Mori-Nu Silken Tofu. All are 100% natural.

Berrilicious

1 cup vanilla soy milk
1/2 cup fresh or frozen strawberries
1 medium banana
1 scoop Vanilla JuicePlus+® Complete or egg white or soy protein powder
4 ice cubes

❶ Blend in Vita-Mix or blender until smooth. Enjoy!

<Makes 1 serving>

▼

If you like berries, you will love this smoothie. If you don't like berries, try this smoothie anyway...maybe you'll change your mind. The more we learn about berries, the better they are for you.

Choco-Mania

1 cup vanilla soy milk
1 scoop chocolate JuicePlus+® Complete
or other chocolate protein powder
1 medium banana
4 ice cubes

❶ Blend in Vita-Mix or blender until smooth. Enjoy!

<Makes 1 serving>

▼

This is the chocolate lovers delight. Add more ice to make it thick and cold like a real smoothie.

Chocolate Delight

1/2 cup old fashioned oatmeal
1 cup vanilla soy milk
1 scoop chocolate JuicePlus+® Complete or other chocolate protein powder
1 medium banana
4 ice cubes

❶ Blend in Vita-Mix or blender until smooth. Enjoy!

<Makes 1 serving>

▼

If you haven't figured it out by now, I love oatmeal, so naturally this is my very favorite smoothie. I have one of these everyday. If you're doing a lot of weight training, add an extra scoop of pure protein powder like the Jay Robb Egg White.

Mango Mania

1/2 cup chopped fresh or frozen mangos
1 cup soy milk
1 medium banana
1-2 scoops Vanilla JuicePlus+® Complete or other protein powder
4-6 ice cubes

❶ Combine all ingredients in a blender and blend until smooth.

❷ Enjoy!

<Makes 1 serving>

▼

This is my all time favorite smoothie recipe! There are a lot of protein powders on the market; however, I think the JuicePLus+® Complete is the best tasting "meal replacement" I have ever tried; I use it in my shakes everyday. One scoop is sufficient for most women. Men and very athletic women should use 2 scoops. If you're an athlete or bodybuilder, do what I do…combine 1 scoop of the JuicePlus+® Complete with 1 scoop of your favorite low-carb, low sugar egg white or whey protein powder for a complete nutritious meal!

The Energizer

1 cup plain non-fat yogurt
1 medium banana
1/2 cup frozen or fresh berries
1 scoop vanilla JuicePlus+® Complete or other vanilla protein powder
4 ice cubes

❶ Blend in Vita-Mix or blender until smooth. Enjoy!

<Makes 1 serving>

▼

This is the perfect post-workout meal. Now that I think about it, it's not bad at just about any time of day.

Strawberry Banana Tofu Shake

1 10.5 oz pkg. Mori-Nu Silken Tofu (soft) (or other soft tofu)
1/2 cup fresh or frozen strawberries
1 medium banana
1 cup vanilla soy milk or orange juice
4 ice cubes

❶ Blend in Vita-Mix or blender until smooth. Enjoy!

<Makes 1 serving>

▼

Ladies, don't forget that soy is very good for your health. Men too. Remember, tofu by itself has no taste, therefore it will taste like whatever you add to it. In this case, it makes a very creamy strawberry-banana smoothie. A number of my busy female clients have this for breakfast every morning.

Mocha Man

1 cup Vanilla Soy Milk
1 scoop Chocolate JuicePlus+® Complete or other chocolate protein powder
1 tsp. instant coffee
1/4 tsp. Vanilla Extract
1/4 tsp. Cinnamon
1 tsp. Honey
4 ice cubes

❶ Blend in Vita-Mix or blender until smooth. Enjoy!

<Makes 1 serving>

▼

Again, if you like coffee, why not make a shake that tastes like coffee. You don't have to use a lot of it. Don't forget, a little bit of hell makes heaven taste mo-better!

The Goddess Nectar

CONTRIBUTED BY BEVERLY MORGAN — SAN JOSE, CALIFORNIA

2 cups soy milk
1 banana
1 nectarine
1 cup frozen cherries or blueberries

❶ Blend in Vita-Mix or blender until smooth. Enjoy!

<Makes 1 serving>

▼

Thank you Beverly from San Jose, California for submitting her favorite quick recipe!

CHICKEN, STEAK, TURKEY & TUNA

NOTE 1: Meats always taste better when they are marinated overnight or at least allowed to sit for 3 to 4 hours in the refrigerator.

NOTE 2: Most of these recipes would also go very well with steamed brown rice. Of course you can't make brown rice in 10 minutes; therefore, I would recommend when you have the time to cook a pot of rice and keep it in the refrigerator. You can then reheat a bowl in the microwave to go with any of the following recipes.

Steak & Asparagus Stir-Fry

1 cup fresh asparagus
1 tbsp. extra virgin olive oil
2 green onions, sliced
1 tsp. fresh ginger
1 tsp. low sodium soy sauce or Bragg's Liquid Aminos
1 tsp. cornstarch
1 cup low sodium beef broth
1 tsp Dijon mustard
8 oz top sirlion thinly sliced

1. Marinate steak in a bowl with soy sauce or Liquid Aminos.
2. Heat oil in skillet over medium high temperature, then add steak.
3. Cook steak for 2-3 minutes.
4. Add asparagus and onions, stir-fry for another 2 minutes.
5. Stir in ginger and mustard.
6. Mix cornstarch and chicken broth together in a bowl then add to skillet.
7. Stir mixture for a few seconds, then let simmer for 1 minute over high temperature.
8. Remove and Serve!

<Makes 1-2 servings>

▼

I used to love this recipe when I was in college. I haven't eaten steak since, but if you like it, this is a very simple and tasty recipe.

Dijon Chicken & Broccoli

1/4 cup low sodium soy sauce or Bragg's Liquid Aminos
1/4 cup rice-wine vinegar
2 tbsp. extra virgin olive oil
2 tbsp. Dijon mustard
1/2 tsp. crushed red pepper flakes
4 cloves garlic, chopped
1 8 oz. skinless, boneless chicken breast
1 cup broccoli, chopped

❶ Combine soy sauce or Liquid Aminos, vinegar, mustard and pepper in a bowl.

❷ Cut chicken into thin slices and marinate in mixture.

❸ Add oil to skillet and heat over medium high temperature.

❹ Stir in garlic for about 10 seconds then add chicken mixture and stir-fry for 3 minutes.

❺ Add broccoli and stir-fry for another minute.

❻ Remove and serve.

<Makes 1-2 servings>

▼

Like most of my recipes, this one came about through experimentation. When you cook as often as I do, you learn to take risks and try new flavors and new combinations. 95 percent of the time I'm very happy with the results, maybe you will be too. (We won't talk about the other 5%.)

Tuna with Tomato & Avocado Salad

1 small avocado, chopped
1 medium tomato, chopped
1 can white albacore water packed tuna, drained
1 tsp. extra virgin olive oil
1 tsp. Dijon mustard
1 tsp. sweet rice wine vinegar
1 tsp. lemon juice
1/4 tsp. thyme
Mrs. Dash to taste

❶ Combine ingredients in a bowl and mix together.

❷ Serve over a bed of baby spinach or mixed greens.

<Makes 1-2 servings>

▼

This recipe was born out of pure necessity. I got tired of eating chicken and egg whites before my bodybuilding contests and fish wasn't always convenient to have around. The combination of tomato, avocado and lemon makes tuna much less boring.

Turkey Breast Fillets with Red Pepper Sauce

8-oz. turkey breast fillets
2 tbsp. tamari sauce
3 cloves garlic, crushed
1 tbsp. Mrs. Dash
2 tbsp. extra virgin olive oil
I medium sized yam, or
1 cup left over brown rice
1 cup broccoli or mixed vegetables

RED PEPPER SAUCE
3-oz. silken soft tofu
1 small red bell pepper, seeded and chopped
4 cloves garlic
1/4 cup vegetable or chicken broth
4 red or green Jalapeno chili peppers
1/2 tsp. organic brown sugar
1/2 tsp. taragon

❶ Cut the yam into small slices and cook in a pot of water over medium-high temperature for 5-10 minutes.

❷ When yam is almost cooked, add the broccoli and cook for 2-3 minutes.

❸ Combine tamari sauce, Mrs. Dash and garlic in a bowl then add turkey breast fillets and marinate well.

❹ Add oil to skillet over medium-high heat. When hot, pan-fry turkey fillets for 1 minute on each side.

❺ While turkey is cooking, combine items for the sauce in a blender and puree for 1 minute.

❻ Pour the sauce over the turkey in the skillet and cook for 1-2 minutes over high heat until sauce is reduced by half. Reduce heat and simmer for another minute.

❼ Serve with broccoli and yam.

<Makes 1-2 servings>

▼

This is one of my very favorite recipes in this book. The sauce is a bit spicy, so feel free to use less of the chili peppers if you can't eat spicy foods. Also, for variety, sometimes you can use chicken or steak fillets instead of the turkey. Enjoy!

Chicken Cacciatora

6 oz. boneless, skinless chicken breast, thinly sliced
6 oz. boneless, skinless chicken thighs, thinly sliced
2 sprigs each of fresh thyme, oregano, sage and rosemary
1 cup dry white wine
6 black peppercorns, crushed
2 tbsp. extra virgin olive oil
1 small can peeled tomatoes, drained
4 cloves garlic, crushed
1 tbsp. tomato paste
1 tbsp. capers (optional)
1/4 cup pitted black olives
1 tbsp. chopped fresh basil
mixed baby salad greens, to serve

❶ Heat oil in skillet over medium-high heat. Sprinkle Mrs. Dash on chicken and stir-fry for 2 minutes.

❷ Add garlic and herbs to skillet and sauté for another minute.

❸ Add the wine, peppercorns, tomato paste and tomatoes to skillet. Cover and simmer for 5-6 minutes over medium heat.

❹ Add capers and olives to skillet and cook uncovered for another minute over high heat, stirring frequently.

❺ Serve with mixed baby salad greens; sprinkle basil on top.

<Makes 2-3 servings>

▼

This is a very simple and healthy way of making a very popular Italian favorite. Whenever possible, always use fresh herbs. If fresh herbs are not available, dry herbs will do just fine.

Veal Fillets with Kiwi, Oregano & Balsamic Vinegar

8-oz. veal fillets, thinly cut to about 1/8 in thick
1 kiwi fruit
2 tbsp. extra virgin olive oil
4 tbsp. balsamic vinegar
1/2 tsp. organic brown sugar
2 tbsp. chopped fresh oregano
1 cup cooked whole grain pasta
green salad

1. Blend kiwi with 2 tbsp. water in a blender until smooth.
2. Place veal in a bowl and prick all over with a fork. Pour blended kiwi fruit over the veal and coat well.
3. Heat oil in skillet.
4. Pat veal fillets dry with paper towel and add to skillet. Cook for 2 minutes on each side.
5. Mix vinegar, sugar and oregano with kiwi marinade.
6. Pour mixture over the veal and cook for another 2 minutes, stirring occasionally.
7. Serve with pasta tossed with 1tsp. olive oil and a green salad.

<Makes 1-2 servings>

▼

If you have time, I would recommend marinating your meats and letting them sit overnight in the refrigerator. It makes the meat more tender and flavorful. Enjoy!

Chicken, Avocado & Rice Salad

2 cups left-over brown or wild rice
2 left-over chicken breasts, cut into small bit-sized pieces
1 ripe avocado, diced
1 lemon, squeezed
2 scallions, chopped
2 tbsp. rice wine vinegar
1 tbsp. balsamic vinegar
1 tsp. extra virgin olive oil
2 cloves garlic, minced
1/2 cup cherry tomatoes, cut in half

❶ Add lemon juice, rice wine vinegar, oil, balsamic vinegar and garlic to a small container and mix well.

❷ Add chicken, rice, avocado and scallions to a large bowl and mix together.

❸ Pour dressing over rice mixture and toss well.

❹ Garnish with tomatoes and serve.

<Makes 2-3 servings>

▼

It's Friday night. You have left-over chicken and rice in the refrigerator and you can't stand to eat chicken breasts one more night, but you also don't feel like cooking. Alas and alack, what do you do? Toss it all in a bowl and voila! ENJOY!

Ground Chicken with Garlic, Basil & Onions

8 oz. extra lean ground chicken breast
4 cloves garlic, minced
1 tsp. dried basil or 2 sprigs fresh basil
1 medium onion, chopped
2 tbsp. extra virgin olive oil
2 tbsp. Bragg's liquid amino or low sodium soy sauce
2-4 red chilies, chopped or 1 tsp. red pepper flakes
2 tbsp. fish sauce
1/4 tsp. organic brown sugar
1 medium-size baked yam
1 cup steamed mixed vegetables

❶ Add 1 tbsp. oil to large non-stick skillet over medium-high heat.

❷ Add 1 tbsp. oil to skillet then add the chicken. Cook chicken for 2-3 minutes, stirring frequently.

❸ Add chili, onion and garlic and sauté for another 30 seconds.

❹ Add basil, fish sauce, sugar and liquid amino and cook for another 3-4 minutes, stirring frequently.

❺ Serve with a salad and baked yam.

<Makes 1-2 servings>

▼

When you buy ground chicken or turkey, always look for the extra lean brand. Or do what I do: buy the skinless breasts from a meat shop and have them ground up. Sometimes I mince them myself in my vitamix machine.

Sweet Tuna Pasta salad

1 cup whole wheat pasta
2 cans white albacore water-packed tuna, drained
1/3 cup chopped celery
1/2 red onion, chopped
1 tbsp. balsamic vinegar
1 tbsp. extra virgin olive oil
2 cloves garlic, minced
2 tsp. Dijon mustard
fresh ground pepper & salt to taste

❶ Cook pasta according to package directions, drain and cool.

❷ Add all other ingredients in bowl with cool pasta and mix together.

❸ Serve over a bed of baby greens.

<Makes 1-2 servings>

▼

This is a very simple, yet quite delicious recipe. Make several servings and keep it in your refrigerator. It tastes great hot or cold. Sometimes I add a little curry powder for variety.

Chicken & Vegetable Stir-fry

6 oz. boneless, skinless chicken breast strips
6 oz. boneless, skinless chicken thigh strips
1 bunch scallions, chopped
1 red bell pepper, sliced
1 small zucchini, chopped
1/2 cup snow peas or sugar snap peas
1/2 tsp. ground turmeric
1/2 tsp. fresh ground ginger
1 tsp. ground cumin
1 tsp. ground coriander
1 tbsp. lime juice
1 tbsp. honey
1/2 tsp. freshly ground black pepper
3 tbsp. olive or canola oil

❶ Combine the turmeric, ginger, pepper, cumin and coriander in a bowl and mix well.

❷ Add chicken strips to mixture and coat thoroughly.

❸ Heat 2 tbsp. of oil in large skillet or wok over medium-high heat.

❹ Stir-fry the chicken until golden brown. Remove and set aside.

❺ Add another tablespoon of oil to the skillet. Stir-fry the vegetables for 2-3 minutes.

❻ Return the chicken to the skillet. Add lime juice and honey and cook for another minute.

❼ Enjoy.

<Makes 2-3 servings>

▼

The aromatic blend of spices makes this chicken dish very special. If you can't find chicken strips at your local market, buy the breast and thigh meat and cut them into bite-sized pieces.

Egg-White Salad Open-faced Sandwiches

6 hard-boiled eggs
1 small avocado, chopped
1 tsp. Dijon mustard
2 slices whole wheat bread, toasted
2 tbsp. fresh salsa

❶ Cut eggs in half length-wise and remove the yolks.

❷ Place egg whites mustard, avocado and salsa in a bowl and mash with a fork.

❸ Sprinkle with pepper and serve over a slice of toast.

<Makes 1-2 servings>

▼

This is a very easy recipe to make. Keep some hard-boiled eggs in your refrigerator at home or at work and make this as a simple mid-afternoon meal. I sometimes use whole wheat tortillas instead of the bread. You can also try the same combination of mustard, avocado and salsa as a topping for your baked potato.

White Bean Turkey Chili

8 oz. ground turkey
1 can white beans
1 medium jar salsa (16 oz.)
1 small can diced pineapples, drained
1 tsp. tomato paste
2 tbsp. cumin
2 tbsp. extra virgin olive oil
1 cup chicken or vegetable broth
1 tbsp. mixed Italian herbs
1 tsp. chili powder
4 gloves garlic, minced
Mrs. Dash
Salad greens

1. Sprinkle turkey with Mrs. Dash.
2. Add oil to skillet over medium heat and sauté garlic, herbs and chili powder for 1 minute.
3. Place all ingredients in saucepan over medium heat and cook for 5-7 minutes.
4. Remove and serve with a salad. Add more Mrs. Dash to taste.

<Makes 2-3 servings>

▼

Again, if you buy the pre-packaged ground turkey, be sure to get the extra lean brand.

Steak with Bourbon Glaze

8 oz. top sirloin steak
3 tbsp. Dijon mustard
3 tbsp. bourbon
1/4 cup low sodium soy sauce or Braggs Liquid Aminos
1/2 tsp. brown sugar
1 tbsp. Worcestershire sauce
1 cup asparagus
1/2 cup vegetable or beef broth
1/2 tsp. cornstarch
1 tbsp. extra virgin olive oil
salt and pepper to taste
1 medium-sized baked potato
salad greens

❶ Cut steak into small bite-size cubes and season with salt and pepper.

❷ In a separate bowl, combine bourbon, mustard, soy sauce, sugar and Worcestershire sauce then add steak. Marinate well.

❸ Heat oil in a skillet and cook steak until brown on all sides.

❹ Add cornstarch and the vegetable broth to left-over marinate; mix together with a fork then add to skillet.

❺ Add asparagus to skillet. Reduce heat and simmer for 5 minutes.

❻ Serve with baked potato and a green salad.

<Makes 1-2 servings>

▼

The combination of bourbon and Worcestershire sauce gives this dish a very unique flavor. Substitute chicken for steak if you don't eat beef. You can bake the potato in the microwave for 5-10 minutes or cut it into small pieces and boil it in a saucepan with water.

Spicy Tuna Salad

By Mardi Luja`n

2 cans white albacore tuna, drained
1/4 cup chopped cilantro
1/2 cup Pace Picante Sauce (Medium hot) or your favorite salsa
2 tbsp. Latin Mayonnaise
(Or 2 tbsp. Nayonnaise and 1 tbsp. finely chopped chili peppers)
1 lime, juiced
mixed greens

❶ Combine all ingredients (except mixed greens) in a large bowl and mix thoroughly.

❷ Serve over a bed of mixed greens.

<Makes 2-3 servings>

▼

This is absolutely the best-tasting tuna I have ever had. The combination of the Latin Mayonnaise and the Picante sauce gives it a creamy and slightly spicy taste. You've got to try it. Mardi runs the Angel City Deli at my gym, Angel City Fitness Center, in Marina Del Rey, CA, and she's a great cook. The next time you're in the area, drop in and have a meal.

Ginger Sesame Chicken

2 tbsp. reduced sodium soy sauce
1 tbsp. minced or grated fresh ginger
3 tbsp. Asian sesame oil
3 cloves garlic, minced
8 oz. chicken breast
1/4 cup chicken stock
3 scallions, chopped
1/2 tsp. corn starch
1 medium baked yam or 1 cup left-over brown rice
1 cup chopped green beans

1. Cut chicken into small bite-size chunks
2. Combine soy sauce, ginger, 1 tbsp. sesame oil and garlic in a bowl then add chicken and marinate.
3. In a skillet, add 1 tbsp. oil and sauté garlic, ginger and scallions for 1 minute over medium high heat.
4. Add another tablespoon oil to the skillet. Add chicken and stir-fry for 2-3 minutes until all sides are brown. Add green beans and stir-fry for another minute.
5. Combine cornstarch and chicken stock in a bowl and mix well with a fork. Pour mixture into the skillet and let simmer for 2-3 minutes, stirring well.
6. Remove and serve with baked yam or left over brown rice.

<Makes 1-2 servings>

▼

Welcome to the orient. Ginger is widely used in Chinese cooking for its health-enhancing benefits. It combines very well with chicken, fish and steak. Enjoy!

Grilled Southwest Chicken Salad with Chili & Lime Dressing

2 boneless, skinless chicken breasts, cut into 1/8″ thick fillets
2 cups mixed salad greens
2 large chopped tomatoes
1/2 onion, diced
2 cups black beans
4 avocado slices
1 tsp oregano
1/2 tsp. chili powder
1/2 tsp. cumin
2 sprigs cilantro

DRESSING

2 tbsp. rice wine vinegar
1 tbsp. flax seed oil
1 tbsp. extra virgin olive oil
4 fresh-squeezed limes
1/4 cup finely chopped cilantro
1 tbsp. finely chopped green chilies
1 tsp. brown sugar
I finely minced green onion

1. Preheat the grill.
2. With a mallet or can, flatten chicken then season it with oregano, chili powder and cumin.
3. Cook chicken over a grill, 2-3 minutes per side, pressing on it occasionally.
4. Toss salad greens, tomatoes and onions and arrange on a plate.
5. Heat beans in microwave then toss over salad.
6. Cut chicken into thin strips and place over salad. Garnish with avocado and cilantro sprigs.
7. Combine dressing ingredients in a container and mix together.
8. Drizzle dressing over salad evenly.
9. Serve and enjoy!

<Makes 1-2 servings>

▼

This recipe may take a little longer than 10 minutes to prepare; however, it's worth it!

Tequila Lime Chicken

2 6-oz. skinless, boneless chicken breasts, cut into thin fillets
1/3 cup tequila
1 tbsp. honey
1 lime (grated zest and juiced)
1/2 tsp. ground cumin

❶ Preheat your oven broiler. Pound chicken breasts flat with a mallet.

❷ Combine tequila, honey, lime juice and zest and cumin in a bowl. Add the chicken and coat well.

❸ Broil chicken but make sure it is at least 4-5 inches from the heat, basting several times with the sauce until chicken is browned outside and white in center…3-4 minutes on each side.

❹ Serve over a bed of baby spinach or mixed greens.

<Makes 1-2 servings>

▼

This dish reminds me of the little tacos I've had in Mexico. Don't worry, the only way you could get drunk from this is if you drank the rest of the tequila in the bottle. The alcohol burns off.

Sesame Lamb with Scallions

8 oz. lamb neck fillet, shredded
2 tbsp. rice wine or dry sherry
2 tbsp. reduced sodium soy sauce or Bragg's Liquid Aminos
1/2 tsp. peppercorns, crushed
3 tbsp. sesame oil
2 cloves garlic, sliced
4 scallions, cut into 1-inch length
1/2 tsp. organic brown sugar
salt and pepper to taste
1 cup chopped fresh spinach
1 cup left-over brown rice

❶ Add lamb, half the soy sauce, 1 tbsp. red wine and peppercorns to a bowl and mix well.

❷ Combine the remaining rice wine, sugar, soy sauce and 1tbsp. sesame oil in a bowl and set aside.

❸ Add the remaining oil to a skillet over medium-high heat.

❹ Add garlic and sauté for 30 seconds then add lamb and stir-fry for 1 minute. Add scallions and cook for another minute.

❺ Stir the sauce into the skillet and simmer for another minute.

❻ Steam spinach with 1/2 cup water in a saucepan over medium heat for 1-2 minutes.

❼ Serve lamb with spinach and left-over brown rice.

<Makes 1-2 servings>

▼

If possible, marinate the lamb and let it sit in the refrigerator overnight.

Del's Almost-World Famous Chicken Curry

2 8oz. boneless, skinless chicken breasts or thighs
2 tbsp. extra virgin olive oil
2 tbsp. Indian curry powder
1/4 tsp. chopped red chili pepper
4 garlic cloves, crushed
1 small onion, chopped
1/4 tsp. organic brown sugar
3-oz. soft tofu
1 small lime, juiced
1/2 cup chicken stock
Mrs. Dash
1 cup left-over brown rice
salad greens

❶ Cut chicken into strips. Put in a bowl with half the lime juice and Mrs. Dash. Marinate well.

❷ Add oil to skillet over medium-high heat then add onion, chili pepper and garlic and sauté for 1 minute.

❸ Add chicken and stir-fry until tender and golden brown. Stir in curry powder and a pinch of salt and stir well.

❹ Add tofu and chicken stock to blender and puree until smooth.

❺ Add puree, sugar and remaining lime juice to skillet. Add Mrs. Dash to taste, reduce heat and simmer for 5-7 minutes.

❻ Serve with left-over brown rice and a salad.

<Makes 1-2 servings>

▼

I learned to make this dish from my grandmother as a young boy growing up in Jamaica. This is my version of a very popular Jamaican dish. Try it and "Welcome to Jamaica, mon!" By the way, in most of my recipes, I use Mrs. Dash as a substitute for some of the salt and pepper the recipe would need. If you can't find it, use a little more salt and pepper.

Garlic Chicken with Green Onions

2 6-oz. boneless, skinless chicken breasts
4 cloves garlic
2 medium-size green onions
1 sweet red bell pepper
1 tbsp. Worchestershire sauce
1 tsp. mixed herb blend
1 tbsp. extra virgin olive oil
Medium-sized baked potato or yam
Mrs. Dash

❶ Cut chicken into small bite-size pieces.

❷ Cut garlic, bell pepper and onions and set aside.

❸ Marinate chicken in a bowl with Worcestershire sauce and mixed herb blend.

❹ Add oil to a skillet and stir-fry chicken for 3 minutes on medium-high heat until brown.

❺ Stir in garlic, onion and pepper and cook for another minute. Add Mrs. Dash to taste.

❻ Remove and serve with a small baked potato or yam.

<Makes 1-2 servings>

▼

This dish is very simple yet DELicious! I sometimes add green beans or broccoli for variety.

Hoisin Beef & Broccoli Stir-Fry

1 cup cooked left-over brown rice
8 oz. top sirloin cut into strips
1 tbsp. dry sherry
1 tsp. reduced sodium soy sauce or Bragg's Liquid Amino
1 tsp. cornstarch
2 tbsp. dark sesame oil
Juice from 1 orange
2 tbsp. hoisin sauce
1 tbsp. honey
1 cup broccoli

❶ Combine the beef, sherry and soy sauce in a bowl.

❷ Heat oil in skillet over medium-high heat. Add the beef and stir-fry for 2 minutes.

❸ Add broccoli and stir-fry another minute.

❹ Mix together orange juice and cornstarch and add to skillet.

❺ Add hoisin sauce and honey.

❻ Reduce heat, cover and cook for about 2-3 minutes until beef is cooked through.

❼ Remove and serve with left-over brown rice.

<Makes 1-2 servings>

▼

Hoisin sauce and sesame oil give this dish its oriental flavor. You can find both of these in the Asian foods section of any large supermarket or Asian food store.

Tantalizing Turkey Tacos

Cooking spray
1/2 medium onion, chopped
1/2 green bell pepper, chopped
3 cloves garlic, minced
1/2 tsp. Chili powder
1/2 tsp. Ground cumin
3/4 cup prepared salsa
8 to 12 oz. extra lean ground turkey
4 (7) inch soft whole wheat tortillas
1 avocado, chopped

1. Coat large non-stick skillet with cooking spray over medium-high heat.
2. Add onion, green pepper and garlic; cook for 1 minute, stirring occasionally.
3. Crumple turkey into skillet; sprinkle with chili and cumin. Cook for 2 minutes, stirring frequently.
4. Add salsa; simmer 5 minutes or until sauce thickens.
5. Spoon mixture into tortillas and top with avocado.

<Makes 2-3 servings>

▼

Turkey tacos are very simple to make. Substitute fish instead of the turkey for variety.

Spicy Marmalade Chicken

1/2 cup orange marmalade
2 scallions, chopped
1 tbsp. Dijon mustard
juice of 1 lemon
1/4 tsp. red pepper flakes
2 8-oz. skinless, boneless chicken breasts, cut into bite-size pieces
salt and pepper to taste or Mrs. Dash
1 tbsp. extra virgin olive oil
1 cup cut green beans

1. Coat large non-stick skillet with olive oil over medium-high heat.
2. Sprinkle chicken with salt and pepper or Mrs. Dash.
3. Cook chicken until brown on all sides, 2-3 minutes, stirring frequently. Add green beans and cook for another minute.
4. Whisk together the marmalade, scallions, mustard, lemon juice and pepper flakes in a bowl.
5. Add mixture to skillet, reduce heat and simmer for 3-4 minutes.

<Makes 1-2 servings>

▼

Simple and DELicious.

Gingered Chicken Noodles

8 oz. boneless, skinless chicken breast strips
1 large zucchini, sliced then chopped
2 tbsp. olive oil
4 scallions, chopped
1 tbsp. minced or grated fresh ginger
2 tsp. Thai green curry paste
2 cups reduced sodium chicken broth
3 oz. silken soft tofu
4 oz. medium egg noodles
1 tsp. lemon juice
salt and pepper to taste

1. Heat the oil in a saucepan over medium-high heat and cook chicken until golden brown on all sides.
2. Add the ginger and scallions and cook for another minute.
3. Add another tbsp. of oil then add the zucchini and cook for 1 minute.
4. Add the curry paste to the saucepan and cook for 30 seconds.
5. Add tofu and 1/2 cup chicken broth to blender and blend until smooth.
6. Add tofu mixture, broth and noodles to saucepan. Stir well and let cook for 5 minutes or until chicken and noodles are tender.
7. Add salt and pepper to taste and serve.

<Makes 2-3 servings>

▼

Whenever possible, buy the strips of chicken, turkey or beef. Remember that smaller pieces of meats and vegetables cook faster. For this recipe, feel free to add a teaspoon of fish sauce for a more authentic Asian flavor. Also note that I use tofu in all these recipes instead of cream.

Steak & Broccoli with Spicy Chili Sauce

1/2 cup red wine vinegar
1 tsp. Organic brown sugar
2 shallots, minced
1 tbsp. Thai red chili paste
1 clove garlic, minced
1 tsp. Sesame oil
2 tbsp. Canola or extra virgin olive oil
salt and pepper
8-12 oz. top sirloin, cut into strips
1/4 cup vegetable or beef broth
1 cup broccoli
1 medium baked yam or potato

❶ Combine vinegar, brown sugar, shallots, chili paste, garlic, and sesame oil in a bowl.

❷ Sprinkle a dash of salt and pepper on the top sirloin in a separate bowl, then add 1/4 the vinegar, chili paste mixture and coat steak evenly.

❸ Heat oil in a large skillet over medium-high heat until almost smoking.

❹ Add steak, stirring frequently. Cook until done, 3-4 minutes. Add broccoli and cook for another minute, stirring frequently.

❺ Add the remaining sauce mix and broth to the skillet, cover and simmer over medium heat for about 3 minutes.

❻ Serve with baked yam or potato.

<Makes 2-3 servings>

▼

This dish might sound very spicy but it actually isn't too bad. So go ahead and give it a try. If it isn't hot enough for those of you who like it really HOT, use some extra chili peppers. You can either bake the potato in the microwave for 5-10 minutes or cut it up into small slices and cook it in a saucepan with water for 5-10 minutes. Enjoy!

Balsamic Raspberry Chicken

2 6-oz. boneless, skinless chicken breasts cut into strips
2 tbsp. extra virgin olive oil
1/2 cup red onion, chopped
1 tsp. dried thyme
1/8 tsp. salt
2 tbsp. raspberry preserves
1 tbsp. balsamic vinegar
1/4 tsp. ground black pepper
1/4 cup chicken stock
1 cup steamed green beans

❶ Heat 1 tbsp. oil in large skillet over medium high heat.

❷ Add onion and sauté for 1 minute.

❸ Combine thyme, pepper and salt and sprinkle over chicken.

❹ Add 1 tbsp. oil to skillet, add chicken and cook for 2-3 minutes, stirring frequently.

❺ Add raspberry preserves, vinegar and chicken stock to skillet, stirring constantly until preserves melt.

❻ Reduce heat to medium-low and simmer for 1-2 minutes.

❼ Remove and serve with green beans.

<Makes 1-2 servings>

▼

No more boring chicken. Remember, think creatively when it comes to food. You probably have fruit preserves in your refrigerator, so why not add a little to your next recipe for a sweet, fruity taste. DELicious!

Grilled Chicken Breast Salad

2 6-oz. boneless, skinless chicken breasts
2 cups mixed baby greens or baby spinach
1/2 cup red bell pepper strips
Mrs. Dash or salt and pepper
sliced melon

VINAIGRETTE:
1 tbsp. extra virgin olive oil
1 lemon, squeezed
1 tbsp. Worchestershire sauce
1 tbsp. balsamic vinegar
1 tsp. Dijon mustard
1/8 tsp. brown sugar
salt and pepper to taste
2 garlic cloves, minced

❶ Reduce the thickness of the chicken by cutting each breast into 2 thinner pieces.

❷ Sprinkle chicken with Mrs. Dash and grill for 3-5 minutes or until done.

❸ Combine vinaigrette ingredients in a small bowl, stir well and set aside.

❹ Toss greens and peppers in a large bowl.

❺ When chicken is done, cut into small cubes and add to salad bowl.

❻ Pour vinaigrette over salad and toss well.

❼ Serve with a side of melon.

<Makes 2-3 servings>

▼

This is a great summertime or anytime meal. It is very simple to make. You can also make this dish using left-over chicken breasts.

Seared Beef Tenderloin with Red Wine Sauce

8 oz. center-cut of beef tenderloin
2 tbsp. extra virgin olive oil
1 tbsp. Worcestershire sauce
Mrs. Dash
Salt and pepper to taste
6 small red potatoes
baby greens salad mix

SAUCE:

1 cup red wine
2 shallots, peeled and minced
2 cloves garlic, sliced
1 small onion, chopped
1/2 tsp. dry thyme
1/8 tsp. sage
2 Roma tomatoes, diced
1 tbsp. Worcestershire sauce
1/2 cup low-sodium beef or vegetable broth
1 tsp. cornstarch

❶ Bake potatoes in microwave for 3 to 5 minutes, or until done. Or cut them in half and cook them in a saucepan of water on the stove until done.

❷ Sauté onion, shallots, garlic, tomatoes, thyme and sage in a saucepan with a tablespoon of oil for 1 minute, then add wine and bring to a boil.

❸ Bring mixture to a simmer and let volume reduce by 3/4ths.

❹ Cut beef into small strips and marinate with Worcestershire sauce and Mrs. Dash.

❺ Heat a large skillet with olive oil then stir-fry beef until golden brown on all sides.

❻ Mix broth, cornstarch and Worcestershire sauce until smooth.

❼ Stir the cornstarch mixture into the hot sauce. Increase the heat and let the mixture reduce by half.

❽ Season with black pepper.

❾ Top beef with the sauce and serve with red potatoes and a mixed baby green salad.

<Makes 1-2 servings>

▼

Feel free to substitute other meats such as veal or turkey breast with this recipe. It will taste great with any meat. Enjoy!

Del's World Famous Chicken Salad with Dijon Vinaigrette

1/2 roasted chicken, or
12 oz. grilled chicken breasts
1 medium cucumber, seeds removed and diced
1 red bell pepper, de-seeded and diced
1/2 sweet red onion, finely chopped
1 medium tomato, diced
1 medium avocado, chopped

VINAIGRETTE

1 tsp. fresh mint leaves, finely chopped
1 tsp. fresh minced green chili peppers
1 tsp. fresh basil leaves, finely chopped
1 tsp. fresh grated ginger
1 lime, juiced
2 tbsp. Dijon mustard
2 tbsp. balsamic vinegar
1 tbsp. rice wine vinegar
1 tbsp. sesame oil
1/4 tsp. curry powder

❶ Remove chicken from the bone and shred it into small pieces.

❷ Combine chicken and diced vegetables in a medium sized bowl.

❸ Combine items for the vinaigrette in a separate bowl and stir well.

❹ Add the vinaigrette to the salad bowl and toss well.

❺ Enjoy!

<Makes 1-2 servings>

▼

Like most of my recipes, this 1 came about through experimentation. I had a roasted chicken in the refrigerator but I was sick of eating chicken. I went to the market and picked up quite a few vegetables and fresh herbs—more than I've included here—the result was my now famous chicken salad. Why is it famous? Well, let me tell you. I am a personal chef for a couple of my private clients and they loved this salad so much that I have to make it every week.

Please note that for this to be a ten-minute recipe you need to use a pre-roasted chicken or grill the chicken breasts on a quick cooking electric grill.

Szechwan Chicken or Turkey Stir-Fry

1 pkg. turkey or chicken breast strips
1 red bell pepper, cut into small cubes
1 medium-sized onion, chopped
4 cloves garlic, minced
2 scallions, chopped
1 tsp. fresh grated ginger
1/2 tsp. red pepper flakes
1 tbsp. mixed herb blend or Italian herb mix Mrs. Dash
2 tbsp. tamari or low-sodium soy sauce
3 tbsp. extra virgin olive oil
1 tsp. cornstarch
1/2 cup reduced-sodium chicken stock
2 tbsp. dark sesame oil
1 medium avocado, sliced
1 medium yam, baked (optional)
1 cup broccoli

❶ In a medium bowl, combine chicken or turkey with 1 tbsp. sesame oil and sprinkle with Mrs. Dash; stir well.

❷ Heat 1-tablespoon olive oil in a large skillet over medium heat.

❸ Add bell pepper, onion, garlic, scallions, ginger, red pepper flakes and herb mix to skillet and sauté for 1 minute. Add the broccoli and cook for another 30 seconds; remove and set aside.

❹ Add remaining olive oil to skillet over high heat and stir-fry chicken or turkey for 2 minutes or until no longer pink.

❺ Add the vegetable mixture to the skillet.

❻ Combine cornstarch, tamari and chicken stock in a bowl and mix until smooth. Add mixture to skillet.

❼ Stir in remaining sesame oil.

❽ Reduce heat, cover and let simmer for 2-3 minutes.

❾ Serve with avocado slices and baked yam.

<Makes 2-3 servings>

▼

This is another experimentation that my clients were very impressed with. I usually just bake the yam in the microwave; it takes about 7-10 minutes.

FISH AND SEAFOOD

SEAFOOD TIPS:

Like chicken and steak, fish is best when marinated and refrigerated up to 24 hours. However, you don't want to marinate shrimp for longer than 3-4 hours.

Fish is cooked when it begins to turn flaky and opaque. Shrimp will turn pink in color.

Shrimp Sauté

2 tbsp. extra virgin olive oil
1 lb. peeled and de-veined medium uncooked shrimp
2 tbsp. Chinese rice wine vinegar or dry sherry
1 tbsp. cornstarch
1 egg white
2 cloves garlic, minced
3 scallions, chopped
1/2 cup chopped fresh basil
2 cups cherry tomatoes
1/2 tsp. organic brown sugar
2 tbsp. fish stock or water
1 tsp. reduced sodium soy sauce
1 tsp. dark sesame oil
salt and pepper to taste
1 cup broccoli florets

❶ Combine shrimp with a pinch of salt, 1 tablespoon wine or sherry, the egg white and cornstarch in a bowl and mix well.

❷ Heat 1 tbsp. oil in large skillet over medium-high heat.

❸ Add shrimp and cook 2 minutes on each side until lightly golden. Transfer shrimp to a plate.

❹ Add the remaining oil, garlic, scallions and basil to skillet. Sauté for 1 minute.

❺ Stir in the broccoli and cherry tomatoes and cook another minute.

❻ Add the shrimp, sugar, stock or water, soy sauce, salt and pepper to taste and sauté 1-2 minutes.

❼ Add sesame oil and serve.

<Makes 2-3 servings>

▼

This is one of the simplest dishes you will ever make.

Shrimp Scampi

14 large raw shrimp or prawns de-veined
1 tbsp. extra virgin olive oil
3 cloves garlic, crushed
1 tbsp. dried parsley
1/4 cup white wine
salt and pepper to taste

1. Add oil to a large skillet over medium-high heat.
2. Add shrimp and garlic; cook 2-3 minutes, stirring frequently.
3. Add parsley, salt and pepper and wine; cook for 1 more minute.
4. Serve over a bed of baby spinach.

<Makes 1-2 servings>

▼

Try this healthier version of an old favorite. In general, try using a little olive oil instead of butter; never use margarine—remember earlier we talked about the dangers of hydrogenated oils.

Shrimp & Scallops with Asparagus, Mushrooms & Spinach

2 tbsp. extra virgin olive oil
2 cloves garlic, minced
halved
4 oz. shitake mushrooms, sliced
8 oz. fresh spinach
1 cup chopped asparagus
1 tbsp. pine nuts
1/2 cup cherry tomatoes, halved

2 tbsp. chopped fresh basil
8 oz.. large sea scallops, washed and
8 oz.. medium precooked shrimp
1 tbsp. capers (optional)
1/4 cup dry sherry
2 tbsp. lime juice
salt and pepper to taste

❶ Heat 1 tbsp. olive oil in large skillet over medium heat.

❷ Add half the garlic and pine nuts and sauté for 1 minute.

❸ Add other vegetables, except tomatoes, and sauté for 2 more minutes. Remove and set aside.

❹ Add remaining oil and garlic to skillet over medium-high heat. Add scallops and shrimp and quickly sauté for 2-4 minutes or until no longer pink.

❺ Add capers, sherry, lime juice, basil, salt and pepper and sauté for another 2 minutes.

❻ Return vegetables to skillet. Add tomatoes and mix well. Reduce to a simmer for 1-2 minutes.

<Makes 2-3 servings>

▼

A wonderful young lady actually made this for me on our first date. It was DELicious! To save yourself time, buy the sliced mushrooms and fresh garlic in a jar.

Zesty Orange Sole Fillets

1 orange, juiced
1 lemon, zest and juiced
1/4 cup white wine
1 tbsp. extra virgin olive oil
2 6-oz. fillets of sole
4 oz. soft tofu
1/4 cup water
fresh parsley
1 cup steamed broccoli
salt and pepper

❶ Add the oil to a large skillet over medium high heat; add sole when oil is almost smoking; cook 1-2 minutes on each side.

❷ Add orange and lemon juice, wine and lemon zest; turn up the heat to reduce the liquid by half.

❸ Add water and tofu to blender and blend until creamy. Add mixture to skillet.

❹ Add parsley and salt and pepper to taste.

❺ Reduce heat to low and let simmer for 2 minutes.

❻ Serve with steamed broccoli.

<Makes 1-2 servings>

▼

Sole is probably one of the easiest fish to cook. It is very mild and very low in fat.

Herb Salmon Fillets

2 6-oz. salmon fillets
1 tbsp. mixed Italian herb
1/2 tsp. paprika
1/2 tsp. ground black pepper
1 tbsp. extra virgin olive oil
1/2 cup vegetable stock or white wine
3 cloves garlic, crushed
2 medium tomatoes, chopped into small pieces
3 green onions, chopped
Mrs. Dash

1. In a bowl marinate salmon fillets with Italian herb, paprika and pepper.
2. Evenly coat a skillet with oil over medium-high heat, add salmon when skillet is almost smoking and cook 1-2 minutes on each side.
3. Add garlic, tomato and green onion and cook for another minute.
4. Add vegetable stock, reduce heat and simmer for 3-4 minutes.
5. Serve over a bed of mixed baby greens or baby spinach.

<Makes 1-2 servings>

▼

This is one of my favorite ways to cook salmon.

Honey Mustard Snapper

4 oz. soft tofu
2 tsp. Dijon mustard
2 tsp. lemon juice
1 tsp. honey
4 6-oz. snapper fillets
1/3 cup minced fresh chives
1/2 cup water or fish stock
3 cloves garlic
1/2 small onion
non-stick spray
1-2 cups mixed steamed vegetables

1. Preheat the oven to 450 degrees F.
2. Add water or stock, tofu, onion and garlic to a blender and blend until creamy.
3. In a bowl, combine tofu cream, mustard, honey and lemon juice, and stir.
4. Coat each side of the fish fillets with the mixture and place in a baking pan (spray the pan first with non-stick spray). Pour the rest of the sauce over the fish.
5. Sprinkle chives over the fish.
6. Bake 5-8 minutes. Serve with mixed steamed vegetables.

<Makes 1-4 servings>

▼

The combination of honey and mustard is great on fish or even as a salad dressing. Try it sometime.

Lemon-Ginger Trout

2 6-oz. boneless trout fillets
2 tbsp. Bragg's Liquid Aminos or low sodium soy sauce
1/2 cup white wine
1 tsp. fresh grated ginger
1 medium onion, chopped
1 lemon, juiced
1 tbsp. extra virgin olive oil
1 cup steamed vegetables
salt and pepper

❶ In a bowl, combine liquid amino or soy sauce, wine, ginger, lemon juice and onion. Mix well then add fish fillets. Pierce the fish with a fork to help the marinate penetrate throughout.

❷ Add oil to skillet over medium-high heat. Add fish when oil is hot. Let the liquid drain from the fish before adding it to the skillet. Cook for 2 minutes on each side.

❸ Add marinate to skillet and turn the heat to high for 1 minute.

❹ Reduce heat, add salt and pepper, cover and let simmer for 2 minutes.

❺ Serve with steamed vegetables and/or baked yam.

<Makes 1-2 servings>

▼

I don't remember where I came across this recipe. All I remember is that it was quite easy to make. And it is DELicious.

Mustard Baked Salmon with Lentils

1 cup cooked lentils, rinsed (canned is fine)
1/2 medium onion, chopped finely
3 cloves garlic, minced
1 bay leaf
3 tbsp. extra virgin olive oil
1/2 cup vegetable stock
1/4 cup large grain or Dijon mustard
2 6-oz. salmon fillets
1/4 cup coarsely chopped Italian parsley

1. Preheat the broiler.
2. Mix 1 tbsp. olive oil and the mustard and evenly spread over fish fillets.
3. Spray baking pan with non-stick spray then place fillets in pan.
4. Cook for 5-7 minutes until flaky.
5. While fish is cooking, combine lentils, onion, garlic and bay leaf in a pot with 1 tbsp. olive oil and sauté over medium heat for 2 minutes.
6. Add vegetable stock, reduce heat and cover. Let simmer for 3-4 minutes.
7. Stir parsley into the lentils then serve with fish when done.

<Makes 1-2 servings>

▼

Salmon and lentils make such a great combination. You can also use black beans or other beans if you prefer.

Pan-fried Fish Fillets in Chili and Garlic Sauce

8 oz. sea bass or trout fillets
1 tbsp. reduced sodium soy sauce
1 tbsp. rice wine vinegar or dry sherry
2 tbsp. olive oil
1 cup left-over rice or medium baked yam
salad greens

SAUCE
3 scallions, finely chopped
3 cloves garlic, minced
1 tsp. fresh ginger
1 tsp. chili bean sauce or finely chopped Thai chili peppers
1 tsp. tomato paste
1 tbsp. rice vinegar
1/2 cup chicken stock
1 tsp. cornstarch
1/2 tsp. organic brown sugar
1/2 tsp. sesame oil

❶ Combine soy sauce and vinegar in a bowl. Add fish and marinate well.

❷ Add oil to skillet over medium-high heat. When hot, add fish and pan-fry for 1-2 minutes on each side.

❸ Push fish to one side of skillet. Add garlic, scallions, ginger, chili bean paste or chili peppers and sauté for 30 seconds.

❹ Combine cornstarch in a bowl with chicken stock. Add stock mixture, vinegar, sugar and tomato paste to skillet. Bring to a boil and braise fish in the sauce for 4-5 minutes.

❺ Sprinkle with sesame oil and serve with left-over rice or baked yam and a salad.

<Makes 1-2 servings>

▼

You may notice that most of my recipes have either a Caribbean or Asian flavor. That's because I was born in Jamaica and grew up in New York where I spent a lot of time among Chinese people practicing Kung Fu. Anyway, this recipe definitely has a Szechuan flavor to it. You may notice something similar in Szechuan Chinese restaurants with the exception that they use a whole fish. Enjoy; it's DELicious!

Orange-Lemon Pepper Snapper

2 6-oz. skinless snapper fillets
1 lemon, juiced
1/2 orange, juiced
1 tbsp. grated orange rind
1 medium onion, chopped
1/4 tsp. nutmeg
1/4 tsp. ground black pepper
1 cup green beans, steamed

❶ Preheat oven to 450 degrees F.

❷ Spray baking pan with non-stick spray.

❸ Combine lemon juice, orange juice, rind and onion in blender and purée.

❹ Place fish in baking pan and sprinkle with nutmeg and pepper, then add puréed mixture.

❺ Bake for 6-8 minutes or until fish is flaky.

❻ Serve with steamed green beans.

<Makes 1-2 servings>

▼

The combination of orange and lemon juice gives snapper, normally a mild fish, a nice sweet and sour twist. In my opinion, snapper can be rather flavorless unless you do something interesting with it.

Snapper with Mango Salsa

1/2 cup fresh cilantro, minced
1 large sweet onion, minced
1 yellow and 1 green bell pepper, seeded and minced
2 tbsp. extra virgin olive oil
2 cups fresh mango, minced
3 limes, juiced
3 6-oz. snapper fillets

❶ Spray or oil the grill and grill snapper for 4 minutes on each side.

❷ Mix cilantro, peppers, onion and mango in a bowl. Cover and chill.

❸ Combine oil and fresh lime juice and use it to baste the fish.

❹ Spoon salsa over the fish and serve.

<Makes 2-3 servings>

▼

As a boy growing up in Jamaica, mango was always my very favorite fruit, and it still is today. This dish gives you a nice cool flavor of the islands. Cool runnings, mon!

Salmon with Fresh Avocado, Mango, Pineapple Salsa

1/2 cup diced fresh avocado
1 cup diced mango
1/2 cup diced pineapple
1/4 cup diced red bell pepper
2 tbsp. finely chopped fresh cilantro
1 tbsp. orange juice
1/8 tsp. cumin
1/8 tsp. cayenne pepper
2 6-oz. salmon fillets
salt and pepper to taste
1 tbsp. olive oil
1 lemon, juiced

❶ Sprinkle salmon with salt and pepper and grill 3-4 minutes on each side.

❷ Combine oil and lemon juice in a bowl and use mixture to baste fish.

❸ Combine the first 8 ingredients in a bowl, stir and chill in the freezer until fish is ready.

❹ Spoon salsa over fish and enjoy!!!

<Makes 1-2 servings>

▼

Yum, yum!! This is one of my very favorite salsa recipes. This is also a very typical Caribbean salsa. This kind of salsa would go well with any fish. Remember, the sweeter the fruit the more delicious your salsa will be! ENJOY!

Orange Roughy with Tomato and Green Onions

2 6-oz. orange roughy fillets
2 medium tomatoes, chopped
3 scallions, chopped
3 cloves garlic, minced
1 orange, juiced
1 tbsp. extra virgin olive oil
1 tbsp. Braggs' Liquid Amino or reduced sodium soy sauce
1/8 tsp. ground black pepper
1 cup steamed asparagus

1. Marinate fish with pepper and liquid amino or soy sauce.
2. Add oil to a large skillet over medium-high heat.
3. When oil is almost smoky, add fish and cook 3 minutes on both sides.
4. Add scallions, tomatoes and orange juice.
5. Reduce heat, cover and let simmer for 2 minutes.
6. Serve with steamed asparagus, left-over rice or a baked yam.

<Makes 1-2 servings>

▼

This is another one of my experiments. I love orange roughy; it's a tasty but mild fish with lots of flavor. ENJOY!

Asian-Style Sea Bass

3 6-oz. sea bass fillets
3 scallions, chopped
2 tsp. reduced-sodium soy sauce
1 tsp. grated fresh ginger
2 tsp. Asian sesame oil
2 cups left-over steamed rice
1 cup steamed broccoli or asparagus.

❶ Preheat oven to broil.

❷ Cut a 12 x 18 rectangle of foil. Place fish on foil. Top with scallions, 1 tsp. of the soy sauce, ginger and sesame oil.

❸ Fold the foil into a packet, tightly.

❹ Place packet in oven for 6-8 minutes.

❺ Serve with left-over steamed rice and steamed broccoli or asparagus.

<Makes 2-3 servings>

▼

Sea bass is one of my very favorite fish. It is quite delicate and very easy to cook. The combination of soy and ginger is classic Chinese; so, enjoy Chinese IN tonight instead of ordering OUT.

Salmon Burgers

2 egg whites
1 cup cold left-over brown rice
2 cans water –packed salmon
2 tsp. Dijon mustard
salt and pepper to taste
4 tbsp. whole wheat breadcrumbs
1 cup steamed asparagus
non-stick spray
1 lemon

❶ In a bowl, mix together rice, salmon, mustard, salt and pepper. Make sure to drain the salmon first.

❷ Form the mixture into 4 equal size patties.

❸ Coat patties with breadcrumbs.

❹ Over medium heat, evenly coat a large skillet with non-stick spray.

❺ Cook burgers until brown on both sides.

❻ Remove burgers, squeeze lemon juice over them and serve with steamed asparagus.

<Makes 1-2 servings>

▼

My client Mary loves this recipe. It's easy, quick and delicious. Go for a salmon burger when you're tired of beef, chicken and turkey burgers. Besides, it's faster to cook.

Curried Swordfish with Tropical Fruit Salsa

4 6-oz. swordfish steaks
2 lemons, juiced
4 tsp. curry powder
2 tsp. extra virgin olive oil
1 tsp. cumin
1/8 tsp. salt

❶ Combine all ingredients in a bowl, stir well, then add fish and marinate well.

❷ Remove fish from marinate and place on broiler pan coated with non-stick spray.

❸ Broil fish for 3-4 minutes on each side, basting frequently with left-over marinade.

❹ Serve fish with fruit salsa.

Tropical Fruit Salsa

1 cup diced, peeled mango
1/2 cup diced, peeled papaya
1/2 cup diced, peeled cucumber, seeds removed
1/2 cup diced tomatoes
1/2 cup chopped red onions
3 tbsp. finely chopped cilantro
1 lemon, juiced
2 tbsp. finely chopped jalapeno pepper

❶ While fish is cooking, combine all ingredients in a bowl and toss well.

❷ Cover and chill in freezer until fish is done.

<Makes 2-4 servings>

▼

Salsa adds a special little twist to fish. This salsa is both hot and sweet, so it goes quite well in the summer. But if you're in Los Angeles, like I am, where everyday is a summer day, then you can enjoy this delicious dish year round.

A little bit hot, a little bit sweet
Salsa makes this fishy great to eat
A little salsa with your fishy
The perfect summer treat

DELicious Fish Cakes

8-oz. cod or haddock fillets
3 scallions, chopped
2 tbsp. cilantro, chopped
2 fresh green chili peppers
1 tsp. grated lime zest
1 tbsp. honey
2 tsp. lime juice
1 tbsp. Thai red curry paste
2 tbsp. olive oil
2 tbsp. whole wheat flour
salt and pepper to taste

❶ Cut the fish into small chunks and place in blender or food processor.

❷ Add scallions, cilantro, chili, lime juice, honey and zest and a pinch of salt to blender and process until finely ground.

❸ Coat your hands with flour and divide mixture into small cakes.

❹ Add oil to a skillet over medium heat. Pan-fry the cakes for 3-4 minutes on each side.

❺ Enjoy.

<Makes 2-3 servings>

▼

This is a healthier version of a popular dish. Fish cakes are easy to make and can be eaten anytime of the day. I like to eat fish cakes with mashed avocado and salsa . . . tastes great. Enjoy!

Yellowtail Snapper with Rum, Mango, Ginger and Mint

4 snapper fillets
1/8 tsp. sea salt
1/8 tsp. black pepper
1 cup whole wheat flour
1 tbsp. fresh ginger
1 cup diced fresh mango
1/2 cup chopped mint leaves
1/2 cup rum
2 tbsp. olive oil
1 cup steamed vegetables

1. Season the fish with salt and pepper.
2. Lightly dust the fillets with flour, shaking off the excess.
3. Heat half the oil in a skillet then add fish and cook until brown on both sides, approximately 3 minutes on each side. Remove fish and set aside.
4. Add the rest of the oil to the skillet. Add the ginger, mango and mint leaves and sauté for 1 minute.
5. Whisk in the rum and bring to a boil.
6. Add salt and pepper to taste.
7. Spoon sauce over fish and serve with steamed vegetables.

<Makes 2-3 servings>

▼

This is my all time favorite fish dish. The combination of mango, rum and mint is simply to die for! Yellowtail works best, but feel free to substitute other snappers, or even halibut. ENJOY!

Spicy Fish Tacos

Cooking spray
1/2 medium onion, chopped
1/2 green bell pepper, chopped
3 cloves garlic, minced
1/2 tsp. chili powder
1/2 tsp. ground cumin
3/4 cup prepared salsa
8 to 12 oz. snapper fillet, cut into small strips
4 (7) inch soft whole wheat tortillas
1 avocado, chopped

❶ Coat large non-stick skillet with cooking spray over medium-high heat.

❷ Add fish to skillet; sprinkle with chili and cumin. Cook for 2 minutes, stirring frequently.

❸ Add onion, green pepper and garlic; cook for 1 minute, stirring occasionally.

❹ Add salsa; simmer 5 minutes or until sauce thickens.

❺ Spoon mixture into tortillas and top with avocado.

<Makes 2-3 servings>

▼

This is a very easy recipe to make. I like to make fish tacos on those Friday nights when I really don't feel like cooking but I want to have something simple and delicious.

Zesty Halibut with Mint and Dill

2 6-oz. halibut fillets
1/2 cup coarsely chopped fresh dill
6 sprigs fresh mint
1 small shallot, finely chopped
1/2 tsp. grated lemon zest
1 lemon, juiced
1/4 tsp. salt
1/4 tsp. ground black pepper
2 tbsp. extra virgin olive oil
1/2 cup fish or vegetable stock
2 cups steamed cabbage

1. Add 1/2 the oil to a large skillet over medium high heat.
2. Sprinkle fish with salt and pepper and cook for 1-2 minutes on each side.
3. When fish is cooked, add all other ingredients.
4. Turn the heat up to high for 1 minute, then reduce heat and simmer for 1-2 minutes.
5. Serve with steamed cabbage.

<Makes 1-2 servings>

▼

This is a very simple way of making halibut. It's simple enough for a quick meal but also something elegant enough to serve to company.

Salmon Teriyaki

2 6-oz. salmon fillets
2 tbsp. olive oil
1/4 tsp. ground black pepper
1/4 tsp. salt
4 tbsp. teriyaki sauce
1/4 tsp. brown sugar
2 cups steamed spinach

1. Brush salmon with olive oil and sprinkle with salt and pepper.
2. Place fish skin-side down in a hot non-stick skillet and sear for 2-3 minutes on each side.
3. Combine teriyaki and sugar and add to skillet; cook for 1 minute more on each side.
4. Serve with steamed spinach and left-over brown rice.

<Makes 1-2 servings>

▼

In case you haven't noticed, I am a very big fan of making food taste good. Teriyaki is very popular, but the secret to using these sauces is not to drown your fish or chicken in them like they do at most restaurants. All you need is a tablespoon or two. Enjoy!

Grilled Tuna Steaks

1/3 cup white wine
1 tbsp. extra virgin olive oil
2 tsp. dried oregano
1/4 tsp. salt
1/2 tsp. pepper
3 garlic cloves, minced
2 6-oz. tuna steaks
2 cups steamed broccoli

❶ Combine the first 6 ingredients in a bowl then add steaks and marinate well.

❷ Grill or broil for 3-4 minutes on each side.

❸ Serve with steamed broccoli.

<Makes 1-2 servings>

▼

Tuna is a great source of lean protein. Of course, like all of the fish and meat recipes, it will taste much better if you marinate it in the refrigerator overnight.

Garlic Sea Bass with Red Wine

2 6-oz. sea bass fillets
1/4 tsp. salt
1/4 tsp. ground black pepper
4 garlic cloves, minced
2 tbsp. mixed Italian Herb
1/3 cup dry red wine
2 tbsp. extra virgin olive oil
1 cup mixed steamed vegetables

❶ Season fish with salt, pepper and herbs.

❷ Add oil to large skillet over medium heat then add garlic; cook for 30 seconds.

❸ Add fish and cook for 2-3 minutes on each side, until flaky, then remove.

❹ Add red wine and cook for about 2 minutes until sauce is reduced by half.

❺ Remove and serve with mixed steamed vegetables.

<Makes 2-3 servings>

▼

Sea bass is another favorite fish because it is light and flaky. As odd as it might seem to use red wine, it actually complements the garlic flavor of this fish quite well; try a Merlot. Steam your vegetables in a steamer or a medium sauce pan with 1/2 cup water over medium heat while your fish is cooking.

Orange Sesame Swordfish

2 6-oz. swordfish steaks
1/2 cup fresh squeezed orange juice
1 tbsp. lite soy sauce
1/2 tsp. grated fresh ginger
1 tsp. Asian sesame oil
1 cup steamed broccoli

1. Preheat the broiler.
2. Combine orange juice, soy sauce, ginger and sesame oil in a deep bowl.
3. Add fish and marinate well.
4. Remove fish from marinade and place on broiler pan; save the marinade. Broil 3-4 minutes on each side.
5. As fish is cooking, pour marinade in a small saucepan over medium-high heat and cook for 1-2 minutes or until reduced by half.
6. Spoon sauce over the fish and serve with steamed broccoli.

<Makes 2-3 servings>

▼

If swordfish isn't available, you can substitute halibut or tuna.

Grapefruit Ginger Scallops

1 lb. bay scallops
1 tsp. fresh ginger
2 tbsp. olive oil
1/4 cup fruity white wine
1/4 cup grapefruit juice
1 cup cooked left-over brown rice
1 cup steamed vegetables

❶ Combine grapefruit juice, wine and ginger in a large bowl.

❷ Add oil to a large skillet over medium-high heat.

❸ Add scallops and cook for 2-3 minutes, stirring frequently. Remove and set aside.

❹ Add grapefruit mixture to the skillet and bring to a boil over high heat, until sauce is reduced by 1/4.

❺ Return scallops to skillet and cook for another 30 seconds.

❻ Serve with left-over brown rice.

<Makes 1-2 servings>

▼

As I mentioned before, it is always good to have some cooked rice in the refrigerator. Also, for easy preparation, I buy the fresh or froz.en pre-cut mixed vegetables at the supermarket. Enjoy!

VEGETARIAN MEALS

Black Bean Avocado Salad

2 cups left-over cooked brown rice
1 ripe avocado, diced
1 lime, juiced
1 tbsp. extra virgin olive oil
2 tbsp. chopped cilantro
1 can black bean, rinsed
2 scallions, chopped
2 tbsp. rice wine vinegar

❶ Combine all ingredients in a large bowl and toss well.

❷ Serve warm or cold.

<Makes 1-2 servings>

▼

This has always been one of my favorite salads. Another creative way of using left-over rice. It's a good idea to keep extra rice in the refrigerator. (I know I keep telling you this, but I want to make sure you get it!) If you don't have any rice available, pick some up from your local Chinese restaurant.

Tofu Burrito

8 oz. firm tofu, mashed
1/2 cup green peppers, chopped
1 medium tomato, chopped
2 whole wheat (or wheatless) tortillas, toasted
olive oil cooking spray
1 small avocado, chopped
2 green onions, chopped
1/4 cup mild/spicy salsa
Mrs. Dash

❶ Coat skillet with olive oil spray over medium heat.

❷ Sauté tomatoes, pepper and green onions for 1 minute.

❸ Add tofu, Mrs. Dash, and salsa and cook for another minute.

❹ Spoon mixture onto tortillas, topped with avocado, roll into a burrito and enjoy.

<Makes 2-3 servings>

▼

This is a great breakfast meal. If I have successfully convinced you to get away from the 3 meal a day concept, then it is a great any time of the day meal. If you've never tried tofu, give this a try. You'll love it, guaranteed!

Sesame Tofu, Broccoli, Tomatoes & Zucchini

8 oz. extra firm tofu, cut into small cubes
1/2 cup broccoli florets
1/2 cup sliced mushrooms
1 medium zucchini, chopped
1 large tomato, diced
2 tbsp. Bragg's Liquid Aminos or reduced sodium soy sauce
2 tbsp. red wine vinegar
2 cloves garlic, minced
2 tbsp. extra virgin olive oil
1 tbsp. sesame oil
1/4 tsp. red pepper flakes
1/4 cup vegetable broth
1/2 tsp. fresh grated ginger

❶ Add olive oil to large skillet over medium heat.

❷ Sauté tofu until brown on all sides, 1-2 minutes. Remove and set aside.

❸ Add remaining oil to skillet and sauté broccoli, mushrooms, zucchini and garlic for 1 minute.

❹ Add tomatoes and sauté for another minute.

❺ Combine Bragg's, vinegar, sesame oil, ginger and pepper flakes in a bowl, then pour the mixture over the vegetables, stirring.

❻ Return tofu to skillet.

❼ Add vegetable broth, reduce heat and simmer for 2 minutes.

<Makes 1-2 servings>

▼

If possible, I would recommend marinating your tofu in the refrigerator overnight. It is much more flavorful that way. Sesame oil, rice wine vinegar, Bragg's Liquid Aminos and a little olive oil make a great marinade.

Tempeh with Peas and Tomatoes

8 oz.. tempeh, crumbled
1/2 tsp. dried basil
1/2 tsp. oregano
1/4 tsp. anise seeds
3 cloves garlic, minced
1 medium onion, chopped
1 cup peas
1 cup fresh or canned diced tomatoes
1 cup vegetable broth
salt and pepper to taste
2 tbsp. olive oil

❶ Heat half the oil in skillet over medium-high heat. Add tempeh and stir-fry for 2 minutes. Remove and set aside.

❷ Add remaining oil, basil, oregano, anise, onion and garlic and sauté for another minute.

❸ Stir in the peas, tempeh, tomatoes and vegetable broth. Cover and cook for another 2 minutes.

❹ Add salt and pepper to taste and serve.

<Makes 1-2 servings>

▼

Fresh ingredients always work best. However, canned tomatoes and froz.en peas will work just fine. Remember, when you crumble your tempeh, tofu or seitan, they will cook much faster with less oil.

Pan-Fried Tofu with Cucumber Sesame Seed Sauce

12 oz. tofu, drained
2 egg whites and 1 whole egg, beaten
2 tbsp. cornstarch
olive oil cooking spray
2 tbsp. reduced sodium soy sauce
1 tbsp. fresh grated ginger

CUCUMBER SESAME SEED SAUCE:
1 tsp. Chinese dry mustard mixed with 1 tbsp. water
1 tsp. mirin or cooking wine
3 tbsp. reduced sodium soy sauce
1 tbsp. toasted sesame seeds
1 small cucumber, chopped into small pieces, seeds removed

❶ Dry tofu with paper towel then cut into 8 pieces.

❷ Marinate tofu in soy sauce and ginger and let sit in the refrigerator for 2 minutes.

❸ Mix sesame seed sauce ingredients together in a bowl and set aside.

❹ Spray a non-stick skillet evenly with olive oil spray over medium-high heat.

❺ Coat tofu with cornstarch, dip into beaten eggs and pan-fry until golden brown on both sides.

❻ Serve with Cucumber Sesame Seed Sauce or Dijon mustard.

<Makes 1-2 servings>

▼

If you can't find all the Chinese ingredients for the sauce you could just use soy sauce, cucumber and chopped scallions.

Carrot Tofu Scramble

2 medium-sized carrots, shredded
8 oz. extra firm tofu, drained and crumbled
2 tbsp. reduced sodium soy sauce
1 tbsp. extra virgin olive oil
1 tsp. dark sesame oil
2 tbsp. sesame seeds, toasted (optional)

❶ Heat olive oil in a large non-stick skillet over medium-high heat.

❷ Cook carrots for 2-3 minutes, stirring frequently.

❸ Add tofu and cook for another 2-3 minutes, until carrots are soft, stirring frequently.

❹ Add soy sauce and sesame seeds and cook for another minute.

❺ Stir in sesame oil and serve hot.

<Makes 1-2 servings>

▼

I like to eat this with left-over brown rice and a small salad with mixed baby greens and tomatoes. If tofu doesn't normally rock your world, try eating it this way, you might like it! To shred your carrots use the medium-sized holes on your grater. You do know what that is, don't you? If you don't, ask someone at your local supermarket or wherever kitchen supplies are sold.

DELicious Seitan Fajitas

8 oz. seitan, cut into thin strips
2 large whole wheat tortillas, toasted
1 small red onion, chopped
2 cloves garlic, minced
1 red bell pepper, seeded and sliced into strips
2 tsp. tamari sauce
1/2 tsp. chili powder
1 small avocado, chopped
1 small tomato, diced
2 tbsp. mild/hot salsa

❶ Coat non-stick skillet with olive oil spray over medium heat.

❷ Add onion, garlic and bell pepper and cook for 2-3 minutes, stirring frequently.

❸ Add seitan, chili powder and tamari sauce.

❹ Lower the heat and simmer for 2-3 minutes.

❺ Spoon seitan mixture onto tortillas. Top with avocado, tomato and salsa. Enjoy!

<Makes 1-2 servings>

▼

In case you're wondering "what in the world is seitan (pronounced say-than)?". It has been called the "vegetarian wheat meat." Seitan is derived from the protein portion of wheat. It is high in protein and low in fat. You can find this vegetarian meat substitute in all natural food stores and Asian markets. Sometimes I add chopped green chili peppers for a more robust, mouth-watering experience! Take it from ol' Del, now and then, set your mouth on fire. Who knows, you might just like it.

Black Beans, Ginger & Tofu

2 tbsp. olive oil
8 oz. extra firm tofu, drained and cut into 1 inch cubes
1 tsp. fresh ginger
1 cup black beans, drained and rinsed
2 cloves garlic, minced
2 scallions, cut into 1/2 inch length
1 red bell pepper, seeded and cut into small strips
1 tbsp. cornstarch mixed with 1/2 cup vegetable stock or white wine
1 tbsp. Chinese rice wine or dry sherry
2 tbsp. tamari
1 tbsp. Bragg's Liquid Aminos or reduced sodium soy sauce
1/2 tsp. red pepper flakes
2 egg whites, beaten
2 tbsp. cornstarch
salt and pepper to taste

❶ Add the oil to a large skillet over medium-high heat.

❷ Coat tofu with cornstarch, dip into beaten egg whites and pan-fry until golden brown on both sides, then remove and set aside.

❸ Add 1 tbsp. olive oil to skillet. Add black beans, garlic, ginger, scallions and bell pepper. Sauté for 1 minute.

❹ Return tofu to skillet and add rice wine or sherry, tamari, red pepper flakes and Bragg's Liquid Aminos.

❺ Add cornstarch mixture to skillet, stirring constantly until it thickens.

❻ Add salt and pepper to taste.

❼ Remove and serve with left-over brown rice and a small mixed-greens salad.

<Makes 1-2 servings>

▼

In my junior and senior years at Columbia University, I was the R.A. for the 8th floor of McBain Hall. And would you believe this was where I first made this dish for my entire floor? Only, I used chicken. Tofu wasn't very popular with me back then.

Tofu Teriyaki

8 oz. extra firm tofu, drained and cut into 1/2 inch cubes
2 tbsp. reduced sodium soy sauce
1 tsp. brown sugar
2 tbsp. rice vinegar
1 tsp. cornstarch
1/4 tsp. red pepper flakes
2 tbsp. dark sesame oil
1 cup broccoli or mixed vegetables
2 cloves garlic, minced
1/2 cup vegetable broth
1 cup left-over brown rice or quick cooking rice

1. Mix together soy sauce, vinegar, sugar, cornstarch, vegetable broth and red pepper flakes in a small bowl and set aside.
2. Add 1 tbsp. oil to skillet over medium-high heat. Add tofu and cook until brown on all sides. Remove and set aside.
3. Add 1 tbsp. oil to skillet. Add garlic and sauté for 30 seconds. Add broccoli or mixed vegetables and cook for 2-3 minutes, stirring frequently.
4. Return tofu to skillet and stir in soy sauce mixture. Bring to a boil until it thickens.
5. Serve over left-over brown rice or quick cooking rice.

<Makes 1-2 servings>

▼

Notice that I didn't have teriyaki sauce anywhere in the ingredients list. This is because teriyaki is really just a seasoned soy sauce. Try this same recipe with chicken if you're a meat lover.

Curried Tofu Salad Sandwich

8 oz. firm tofu, drained and crushed
2 scallions, chopped finely
1 red bell pepper, chopped finely
1 small carrot, shredded finely
1 tsp. Dijon mustard
1 tsp. rice wine vinegar
1/4 tsp. salt
1/2 tsp. curry powder
1/4 tsp. ground black pepper
2 large whole wheat tortillas, toasted
1 tbsp. chopped fresh parsley
Romaine lettuce

❶ Mix all ingredients together, except tortillas and lettuce.

❷ Spoon mixture over tortillas. Top with lettuce and serve.

<Makes 2-3 servings>

▼

Of course, you can easily replace the tofu with egg whites. You could even use a couple hard boiled egg whites with the tofu. Great combination. Enjoy!

Tomato Basil Tofu Scramble

8 oz. firm tofu, crumbled
1 medium tomato, chopped
2 tbsp. fresh basil, chopped
1/2 medium onion, chopped
2 cloves garlic, minced
1/2 tsp. Italian herb
1 tbsp. extra virgin olive oil
salt and pepper to taste
2 tbsp. mild salsa (optional)
1-2 whole wheat tortilla(s)

❶ Add oil to a large skillet over medium-high heat.

❷ Sauté tomato, onion, garlic and basil for 2 minutes.

❸ Add tofu and scramble for another 2-3 minutes.

❹ Add salsa, salt and pepper to taste. Serve with toasted whole wheat tortilla and a piece of your favorite fruit.

<Makes 2-3 servings>

▼

When I tire of eating eggs, I go for the tofu scramble. For variety, try adding a piece of avocado or even a teaspoon of peanut butter.

Three-Bean Chili with Tofu

8 oz. extra firm tofu, crumbled
1 cup cooked black beans, drained and washed
1 cup cooked red kidney beans, drained and washed
1 cup great northern white beans, drained and washed
1 16-oz. can diced tomatoes
1 medium onion, finely chopped
3 cloves garlic, minced
1 yellow bell pepper, seeded and chopped
2 tbsp. tomato paste
1 tbsp. extra virgin olive oil
1 tsp. chili powder
1/2 tsp. cayenne pepper
1/2 tsp. cumin seeds
1 tsp. dried oregano
1/4 cup chopped fresh cilantro or fresh parsley
1 cup vegetable broth
salt and freshly ground black pepper to taste

1. Add oil to large skillet over medium heat. Add onion, garlic, chili, cumin, cayenne pepper and oregano. Sauté for 1 minute.
2. Add bell peppers and tofu and sauté for another minute.
3. Stir in tomatoes, broth, tomato paste and the beans and bring to a boil.
4. Reduce heat and simmer for another 3 minutes.
5. Season with salt and pepper to taste and stir in cilantro or parsley then serve.
6. Reduce heat and simmer for another 3 minutes.

<Makes 1-2 servings>

▼

This is one of my favorite winter time dishes. It is easy to make and tastes great!

Tofu & Vegetables with Cashews

1 tbsp. light soy sauce or Bragg's Liquid Aminos
1/2 tsp. cornstarch
2 tsp. honey
1 tsp. hot bean sauce
1 tbsp. water
1 tsp. sweet bean sauce
3 tbsp. extra virgin olive oil
1 carrot, chopped
1 zucchini, chopped
12 oz. extra firm tofu, cut in 1/2" cubes
1/2 cup froz.en peas
1/4 cup roasted unsalted cashews

❶ Combine the first 6 ingredients in a bowl and stir until honey and cornstarch is completely dissolved.

❷ Place large skillet over medium-high heat. Add oil when skillet is hot.

❸ Add carrots and stir-fry for 30 seconds.

❹ Add zucchini, tofu, and peas; stir-fry for 1 minute.

❺ Stir in cashews.

❻ Stir in the sauce and stir until thickens, about 1 minute.

<Makes 3-4 servings>

▼

The bean sauce gives this dish a nice Asian flavor. You should be able to find bean sauce in the Asian foods section of most supermarkets.

Spicy Tofu & Asparagus with Garlic Ginger Sauce

2 tbsp. light soy sauce
1/4 cup vegetable stock
1/4 cup green onions, thinly chopped
1 tsp. fresh garlic, minced
1 tsp. minced jalapeno pepper
1 tsp. fresh ginger, minced
1 cup chopped asparagus
8 oz. extra firm tofu, cut in 1/2″ cubes
2 tbsp. extra virgin olive oil
1 tsp. cornstarch
1 tsp. honey

❶ Place large skillet over medium-high heat.

❷ Combine soy sauce, cornstarch and vegetable stock in a bowl and mix until cornstarch completely dissolves.

❸ Add the oil to the skillet. Add tofu and stir-fry for 1 minute then add asparagus and cook for another minute.

❹ Add green onions, garlic, jalapeno, and ginger and sauté for 30 seconds.

❺ Stir in the sauce until it thickens, about 1 minute.

<Makes 1-2 servings>

▼

I love this dish. It is simple and quite delicious. I use a lot of jalapeno, but if you're a spice sissy, feel free to use a little less.

Oatmeal Tofu Pancakes with Applesauce

5 oz. silken light tofu
1/4 cup applesauce
1 cup soy milk
1/4 cup whole wheat flour
1 cup old fashioned oatmeal
2 tbsp. honey
1 tsp. salt
3 tbsp. baking powder

❶ Blend tofu, applesauce, honey and soy milk together in a blender.

❷ Add flour, oatmeal, baking powder and salt together in a large bowl.

❸ Add the blender mixture to the bowl and mix well.

❹ Spray a non-stick skillet (or a griddle) with olive oil base cooking spray over medium heat.

❺ Pour batter onto hot, lightly sprayed griddle or skillet.

❻ Cook until tiny bubbles form on top of pancakes, then turn over (approximately 1-2 minutes on each side).

❼ Serve pancakes hot with fruit preserve or apple sauce.

<Makes 1-2 servings>

▼

If you don't eat eggs, tofu is a great alternative. These are very light pancakes that I sometimes have with a protein smoothie. By the way, don't pour all the batter onto the griddle at the same time. Pour just enough to form a small pancake 4-6 inches in diamcter. In case you slept through high school geomctry, the diameter of a circle is the length across the middle. Enjoy!

Ginger Orange Tofu with Spinach

8 oz. extra firm tofu, cut into 1/2″ cubes
1 cup fresh spinach, chopped
1/4 cup fresh squeezed orange juice
1 tsp. fresh grated ginger
2 tbsp. extra virgin olive oil
2 cloves garlic, minced
3 scallions, chopped
2 tbsp. tamari sauce
salt and pepper to taste

❶ Marinate tofu in a bowl with tamari sauce.

❷ Add oil to a skillet over medium-high heat.

❸ Add the tofu and stir-fry for 1 minute. Add garlic, scallions, and ginger and cook for one more minute.

❹ Add the spinach and stir-fry for another minute.

❺ Pour in the orange juice and bring to a boil, then reduce heat and simmer for 1 minute.

❻ Add salt and pepper to taste and serve.

<Makes 1-2 servings>

▼

Feel free to use both the orange juice and the zest of the orange as well. DELicious!

Tofu & Cabbage with Ginger and Scallions

8 oz. firm regular tofu (not silken), cut into 1/2″ cubes
1 cup green cabbage
2 scallions, chopped
1 tbsp. fresh grated ginger
2 tsp. tamari or light soy sauce
2 tbsp. sesame oil
salt and pepper to taste

❶ Place a large skillet over medium-high heat. Add oil.

❷ Stir-fry tofu, scallion and ginger for 1 minute.

❸ Add cabbage and stir-fry for another minute.

❹ Add tamari sauce, salt and pepper to taste, stir for another 30 seconds then serve.

<Makes 1-2 servings>

▼

Here's another simple tofu idea. This is actually a re-creation of a dish I useD to have at my favorite neighborhood Chinese restaurant. Enjoy!

Lentil Salad

1 can lentils, rinsed and drained
4 hardboiled egg whites, chopped
2 tomatoes, diced
1/2 cucumber, diced
1/2 red onion, finely chopped

VINAIGRETTE DRESSING:
2 tbsp. light soy sauce or Bragg's Liquid Aminos
1 tbsp. Dijon mustard
1 tbsp. rice wine vinegar
1 clove garlic, minced

❶ Combine salad ingredients in a large bowl and toss well.

❷ Combine ingredients for the vinaigrette in a small bowl and mix well.

❸ Pour vinaigrette over the salad and toss well.

<Makes 1-2 servings>

▼

I love lentils. This recipe came about through experimentation on a day I had nothing in my refrigerator but eggs and a can of lentils in the cabinet. It's quite good.

15 QUICK, EASY & VERSATILE TOFU TOPPINGS
For Baked Potatoes, Brown Rice & Other Whole grains

By Marilyn Joyce, MA, RD, Ph.D. (c)
Author — *5 Minutes to Health*
Author — *I Can't Believe It's Tofu!*

1. Equal parts nonfat, plain yogurt and soft tofu blended with chives.
2. Equal parts low fat firm tofu and salsa mashed together.
3. Soft tofu blended until smooth with minced red peppers, ginger and olives.
4. Scrambled egg and shredded extra firm tofu mixture topped with salsa.
5. Firm tofu seasoned with minced garlic, onions, celery and Spicy Mrs. Dash.
6. Low fat soft or silken tofu and almond butter blended with jalapeno peppers.
7. Low fat soft tofu and sardines blended or mashed together.
8. Blended soft or silken tofu, raisins, almonds and hot pepper sauce.
9. Blended broccoli, cauliflower, onions, garlic and soft tofu.
10. Mashed avocado and firm tofu, mixed with chopped tomatoes, onions and garlic.
11. Mashed avocado, firm tofu and spicy salsa mixed.
12. Mashed firm tofu, onions, minced garlic, fresh lemon juice and hot pepper sauce.
13. Soft or silken tofu and apricots blended together and mixed with chopped walnuts.
14. Soft or silken tofu and tahini blended together and mixed with dark raisins.
15. Low fat firm tofu mashed and mixed with chopped prunes and almonds.

Note: Though it is not always written, it must be understood that any tofu used, can be of the low fat or regular variety. These toppings are designed to be high enough in protein to make the baked potato or grain a meal. Just add a salad, with nonfat homemade dressing, to complete the meal.

Today

BY KELLY O'CONNOR
MARINA DEL REY, CALIFORNIA

I do not trust myself.
I do not trust
that I can and will
take care of myself.
This is the issue for me today.

I do what is necessary to get by.
I fudge
and fake it
where I can.
And, I am not proud,
but have a sense of indignant pride
that carries me forward with this pattern.
"This is the way I am."
"This is the way I've always been."
But, I want it to be different.
I want to be different.
I want to feel a motivation
from inside
to love myself
no matter what.
To take care of myself
when it isn't easy.
To be the woman of MY dreams
rather than waiting
on some man
to say that I am his.

Victory is about celebrating
each step along the journey,
and I am stuck.
I don't feel like celebrating today,
and I don't feel like working.
There is so much I feel is wrong,
yet I am better than I ever have been.

Maybe
authenticity
is the victory
for today,
and reaching out
another.
Maybe it is a good day
after all.

Kelly is one of my dearest clients and a very good friend. And as you can tell, she is also a brilliant poet. She is currently working on a book of poetry that is a must read.

Email her your words of encouragement to my attention (del@delmillers.com) and I will forward them to her.

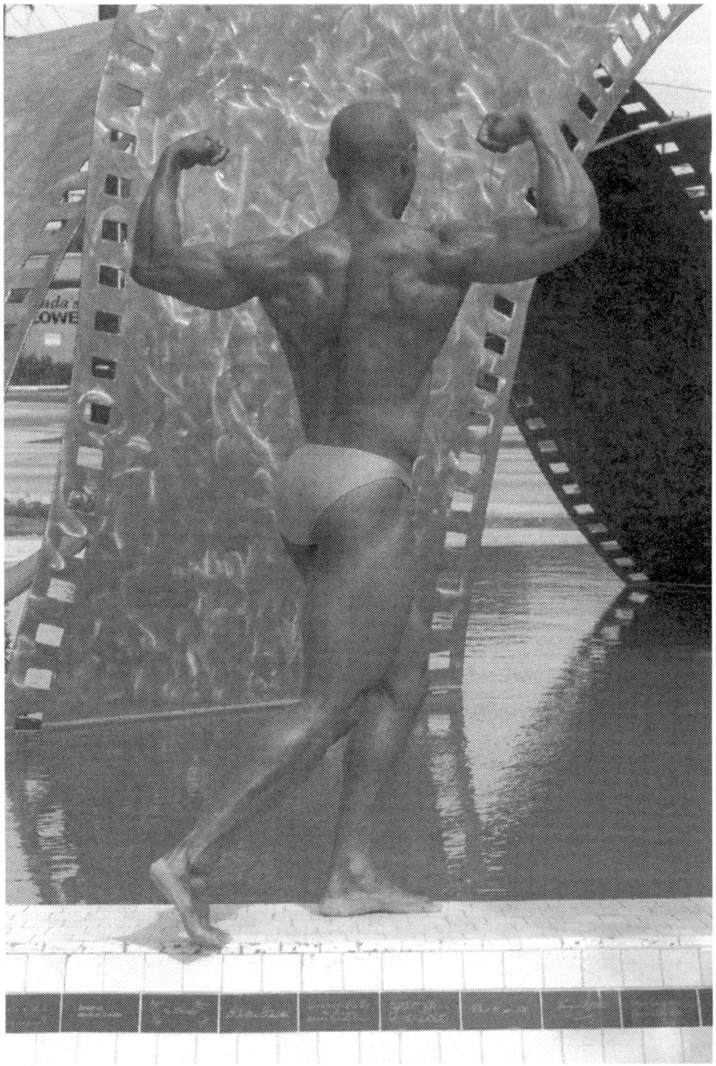

"Start every day with a smile
and get it over with."
— WC Fields

The Stairmaster Blues!*

I'm tired, I'm bored
I'm sticky, I'm sweaty
This is way too hard
Enough already

This sucks, this hurts
I truly hate pain
I look so stupid
This is really insane

I don't want to do this today
Why me?, I've been doing OK
Why am I doing this anyway?

No matter what they try to say
This doesn't feel at all like play
Why am I doing this anyway?

I've been on this thing
Forever again
What time is it now
Never never again!

My feeble mind's on holiday
My butt is tired, my feet are clay
Why am I doing this anyway?

It's only ten minutes?
This is all a bad dream
Get me off of here
I'm about to scream!
I'm About To Scream!!
I'm About to Scream!!!

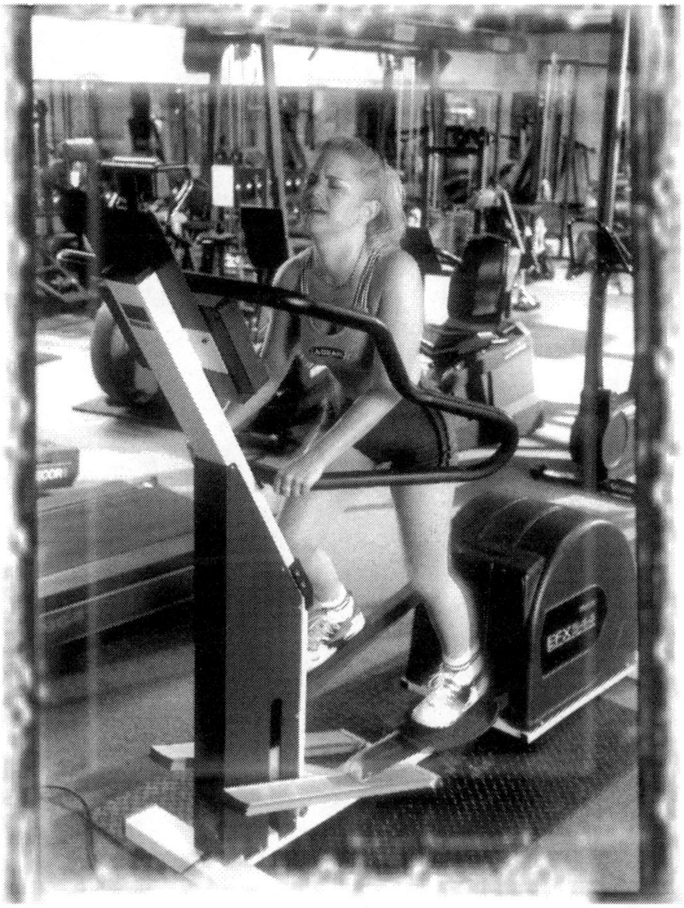

*(Dancing with God - Republished as Fitness & Spirituality, Spiritwind, 2012)

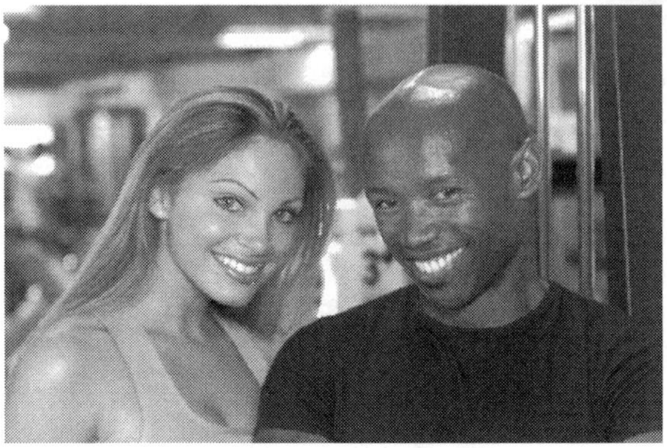

Acknowledgements

I want to express my gratitude to my photographer Michael Burr for his continued support.

Special thanks to my editor, Jack Barnard; my designer, Dotti Albertine; my assistant, Pam Thomas; and my proofreader, Kara Masters; for their creative inputs.

My gratitude also goes to Ellen Reid for her wonderful suggestions. And to my favorite client and friend, Jenny Leone, for gracing these pages with her beautiful smile.

Thanks to all my clients and friends who encouraged me to write this book.

And finally, a very special thanks to Marilyn Joyce, Mardi Luja'n and Beverly Morgan for their recipes. And to Kelly O'Connor for her wonderful poem.

About the Author

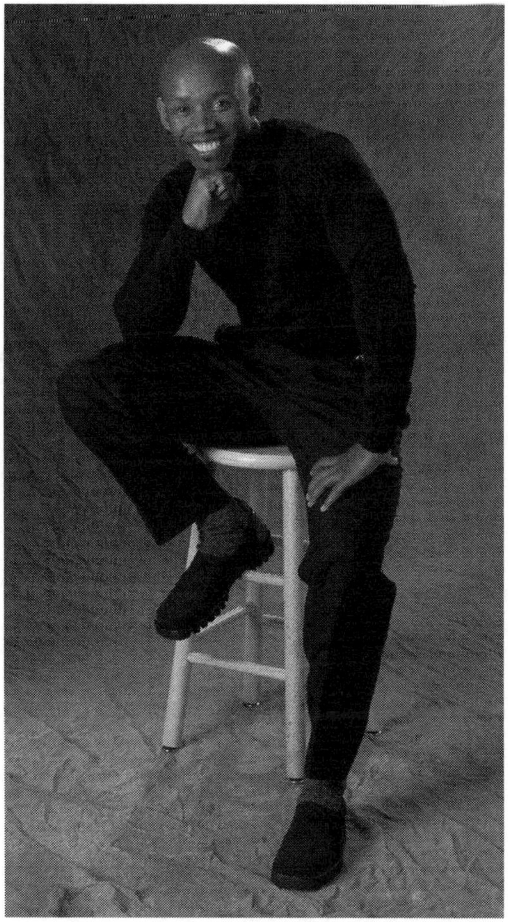

DEL MILLERS, PHD
Author, Speaker, Life Coach

DEL THE AUTHOR

Other Books by Del Millers:

DR. DEL'S RAPID FATLOSS MANUAL:
A Scientific Approach to Building Your Leanest Body Ever

DR. DEL'S RAPID FATLOSS COOKBOOK:
Quick & Easy "10-Minute Meals" for Building Your Leanest Body Ever.

DR. DEL'S RAPID FATLOSS DETOX-CLEANSE PROGRAM:
A 21-Day Whole Food Based Plan for Jumpstarting Your Body's Fat-Burning System.

DR. DEL'S RAPID FAT LOSS MEAL PLAN:
Quick & Easy 10-Minute "Fit" Recipes and Nutrition Guide.

DEL'S 10-MINUTE TOTAL BODY WORKOUT:
When all you've got is 10 minutes to spare!

DANCING WITH GOD:
How you can Make Exercise a Playful Adventure of Body and Soul!

Del The Speaker

SPEAKING ENGAGEMENTS AND SEMINARS:

Speaking the Spirit of the Body's Wisdom

When Del Millers speaks, people listen. He knows an awful lot about the physical body, and he looks like it. He also knows an awful lot about the mind and emotions, and he demonstrates it. And that he has a very intimate and personal relationship with his own spiritual nature puts him in a very unique position to be able to support, motivate, encourage people to reach new levels with their personal dreams and ambitions. As one client puts it, "I have had many personal fitness trainers and many dance and tennis teachers. Del is the first one to really help me reach my goals. He's tough and demanding and kind at the same time. He knows what he's doing; he's an expert."

Del has been extremely successful as a motivational speaker and coach because he addresses all aspects of the human being. He is intelligent, well spoken, and engaging, whether he's exploring the many aspects of health and nutrition or describing how exercise is really like dancing with God. He fascinates audiences and individuals alike because he practices what he preaches. He is a happy man with a firm grasp on his reality—and he assists others to reach the same amazing place. He is, in a word, inspiring.

Del holds a Masters Degree in Spiritual Psychology, a degree he earned by demonstrating self-mastery, and a Ph.D. in Exercise and Nutritional Science. He is also an accomplished writer, poet, and performer as well as a master instructor of Kung Fu and Tai Chi Chuan, a Personal Fitness Coach and a sought after corporate consultant. Del is truly a pioneer, combining the fields of Fitness and Transformation.

Del Millers is a powerhouse, standing on a solid foundation of education and experience. When he speaks, people want what he's got. The good news is, he knows how to deliver.

Private Consultation

Dr. Del is available for phone or email fitness, nutrition and life coaching.

DEL'S CONTACT INFORMATION:

For consultations or to book Del for a seminar or speaking engagement, please contact:

DEL MILLERS
Del Millers International
10736 Jefferson Blvd. #693
Culver City, CA 90230
USA

http://www.delmillers.com
del@delmillers.com
1-888-800-9463

SUBSCRIBE TO DR. DEL'S FREE EMAIL NEWSLETTER:
www.drdelmillers.com

SUBSCRIBE TO DR. DEL'S BLOG:
www.drdelblog.com

DR. DEL'S ONLINE FITNESS & NUTRITION COACHING PROGRAM:
GET A FREE FITNESS ANALYSIS AND ONE-MONTH MEMBERSHIP
www.personalfitness.com

JOIN THE CONVERSATION ONLINE:

FACEBOOK
Facebook.com/drdelmillers
Like Dr Del for daily updates and postings

TWITTER
@drdelmillers
Stay connected

YOUTUBE
Youtube.com/drdelmillers
Visit Dr. Del's video channel

DEL MILLERS INTERNATIONAL

Inspiration, Support & Encouragement,
For Your Personal Growth and Transformation!
http://www.delmillers.com

Made in the USA
Monee, IL
13 September 2026

62979548R10098